The Ultimate Nurse Practitioner Guidebook

"Nadia Santana, DNP, FNP-BC, has created a true masterpiece. As someone who has been professionally active in the nursing profession since 1987, I was not only incredibly proud to read her thoughtful and detailed guidebook, but I learned a lot myself. Dr. Santana's guidebook is essential for anyone who is interested in becoming a nurse practitioner—both those who are already nurses and those who are starting out in the profession. Dr. Santana has beautifully illustrated what makes nurse practitioners a crucial and integral part of achieving quality health care for consumers in the US."

—*Dyan Summers, DNP, ANP-BC, MPH, CTH®Jonas Scholar*
Nurse Practitioner who diagnosed, treated, and reported the first
American recreational traveler to be infected with the ZIKA virus

"*The Ultimate Nurse Practitioner Guidebook: A Comprehensive Guide to Getting Into and Surviving Nurse Practitioner School, Finding a Job, and Understanding the Policy That Drives the Profession* is a wonderful resource for nurses contemplating the nurse practitioner profession and early career nurse practitioners. Nadia Santana, DNP, FNP-BC, presents clear information and offers insightful tips, from helping readers navigate the process of researching schools to securing their first NP position."

—*Stephen Ferrara, DNP, FNP-BC, FAANP,*
Editor-in-Chief, Journal of Doctoral Nursing Practice, *and*
Executive Director, The Nurse Practitioner Association, *NY State*

The Ultimate Nurse Practitioner Guidebook

This book is part of the Peter Lang Education list.
Every volume is peer reviewed and meets
the highest quality standards for content and production.

PETER LANG
New York • Bern • Berlin
Brussels • Vienna • Oxford • Warsaw

Nadia Santana, DNP, FNP-BC

The Ultimate Nurse Practitioner Guidebook

A Comprehensive Guide to
Getting Into and Surviving Nurse
Practitioner School, Finding a Job, and
Understanding the Policy That
Drives the Profession

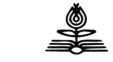

PETER LANG
New York • Bern • Berlin
Brussels • Vienna • Oxford • Warsaw

Library of Congress Cataloging-in-Publication Data

Names: Santana, Nadia, author.
Title: The ultimate nurse practitioner guidebook: a comprehensive
guide to getting into and surviving nurse practitioner school,
finding a job, and understanding the policy that drives the
profession / Nadia Santana.
Description: New York: Peter Lang, 2018.
Includes bibliographical references.
Identifiers: LCCN 2018007995 | ISBN 978-1-4331-5535-2 (hardback: alk. paper)
ISBN 978-1-4331-4927-6 (paperback: alk. paper)
ISBN 978-1-4331-4928-3 (ebook pdf)
ISBN 978-1-4331-4929-0 (epub) | ISBN 978-1-4331-4930-6 (mobi)
Subjects: LCSH: Nurse practitioners—Certification—Examinations,
questions, etc. | Nurse practitioners—Vocational guidance.
Classification: LCC RT82.8.S23 2018 | DDC 610.7306/92—dc23
LC record available at https://lccn.loc.gov/2018007995
DOI 10.3726/b11761

Bibliographic information published by **Die Deutsche Nationalbibliothek**.
Die Deutsche Nationalbibliothek lists this publication in the "Deutsche
Nationalbibliografie"; detailed bibliographic data are available
on the Internet at http://dnb.d-nb.de/.

The paper in this book meets the guidelines for permanence and durability
of the Committee on Production Guidelines for Book Longevity
of the Council of Library Resources.

Printed in the United States of America

DEDICATION

This book is dedicated to all of the teachers, preceptors, mentors, and colleagues who have helped me along my nurse practitioner journey. Thank you for your patience and compassion, and for teaching me how to be the nurse practitioner that I am today.

CONTENTS

VIII THE ULTIMATE NURSE PRACTITIONER GUIDEBOOK

ACKNOWLEDGMENTS

There are so many individuals that I am grateful to for helping me with this book. Thank you to my Acquisitions Editor, Sarah Bode, of Peter Lang Publishing. Without her, this book may never have been finished. A big thanks to both Brittany Pavon Suriel and Dr. Paul Coyne for reading the manuscript in its early version and offering great feedback. Many thanks to Dr. Dyan Summers and Dr. Stephen Ferrara for reviewing the finished manuscript in its entirety. Gratitude and love to all of my wonderful NP friends who have supported me throughout the years. My mother deserves an enormous thank you for reading and rereading my manuscript, many times over. And of course, thank you to my husband Reinaldo, for being so patient and supportive during the numerous months it took to bring this book to life.

PREFACE

Congratulations on making the decision to become a nurse practitioner (NP), one of the most rewarding professions on planet Earth! Whether you have been a nurse for years and have decided to return to school to pursue advanced training or have recently graduated a Doctor of Nursing Practice (DNP) program, choosing to join a group of professionals more than 234,000 strong will change your life in ways you could never imagine.

I wrote this book in order to give you, the reader, guidance about how exactly to become a nurse practitioner. While I was applying to nurse practitioner programs, I found myself lost in the professional jargon that surrounds nursing, and I lacked the understanding of how exactly to become a nurse practitioner. Even with the plethora of internet resources available, I still struggled and was confused about the entire process. I definitely could have used a guidebook to help me along the way, so I created one in hopes of helping future nurse practitioners achieve their dreams. My goal is to assist you every step of the way during this process and also help to make the transition into NP school and then into clinical practice as smooth as possible.

Within these pages you will find an abundance of information on a wide variety of nurse practitioner–related subjects. From how to get accepted into a program, to financing your education, to starting off your practice as a nurse practitioner—we are going to cover it all! Regardless of where you are on your path to becoming an NP, there will be valuable information for you along the way. Even if you are no longer a student, and are already a practicing nurse practitioner, you will still find much of the information presented in this book relevant to your life and clinical practice. Aside from invaluable information about the nurse practitioner profession, I've also included a comprehensive appendix full of helpful references to help you along your nurse practitioner path.

You may find some of the information repeated throughout the text; this is because some of the subjects are very important and I wanted to make sure the concepts are understood. Additionally, at the time of publication the information in this book was correct and up-to-date. As the NP profession continues to evolve and grow, this information may have changed between publication and when purchased. I suggest you do your due diligence while doing your research on NP programs and the profession.

I wish you all the best of luck on your journey to becoming a nurse practitioner. Although the means to actually becoming a nurse practitioner can be at times very challenging, and you may encounter a few bumps along the road, you will also find this profession incredibly fulfilling. With each day bringing new knowledge and professional growth and challenges, rest assured that working as a nurse practitioner will keep you on your toes!

ABBREVIATIONS

- AANP American Academy of Nurse Practitioners
- ACNP Acute Care Nurse Practitioner
- ACPNP Acute Care Pediatric Nurse Practitioner
- AGNP Adult Gerontology Nurse Practitioner
- AGACNP Adult Gerontology Acute Care Nurse Practitioner
- AGPCNP Adult Gerontology Primary Care Nurse Practitioner
- ANP Adult Nurse Practitioner
- ANP Advanced Nurse Practitioner
- AOCNP Advanced Oncology Certified Nurse Practitioner
- APN Advanced Practice Nurse
- APNP Advanced Practice Nurse Prescriber
- APRN Advanced Practice Registered Nurse
- ARNP Advanced Registered Nurse Practitioner
- BC Board Certified
- BSN Bachelor of Science in Nursing
- C Certified
- CE Continuing Education
- CNM Certified Nurse-Midwife
- CNP Certified Nurse Practitioner

- CRNA Certified Registered Nurse Anesthetist
- CRNP Certified Registered Nurse Practitioner
- CNS Clinical Nurse Specialist
- DCNP Dermatology Certified Nurse Practitioner
- DEA Drug Enforcement Administration
- DNP Doctor of Nursing Practice
- ENP Emergency Nurse Practitioner
- FNP Family Nurse Practitioner
- GNP Gerontological Nurse Practitioner
- GPA Grade Point Average
- GRE Graduate Record Exam
- HRSA Health Resources and Services Administration
- ICU Intensive Care Unit
- MSN Master of Science in Nursing
- NNP Neonatal Nurse Practitioner
- NP Nurse Practitioner
- NPI National Provider Identifier
- ONP-C Certified Orthopedic Nurse Practitioner
- PA Physician Assistant
- PCP Primary Care Provider
- PMHNP Psychiatric-Mental Health Nurse Practitioner
- PNP Pediatric Nurse Practitioner
- PNPAC Pediatric Nurse Practitioner, Acute Care
- RN Registered Nurse
- RNP Registered Nurse Practitioner
- SNP School Nurse Practitioner
- TA Teaching Assistant
- WHNP Women's Health Nurse Practitioner

INTRODUCTION

Come dress yourself in love, let the journey begin.

—Francesca da Rimini

The journey for me to become a nurse practitioner was six consecutive years in the making. However, looking back on it, I think I have been on this path my entire life, taking one small baby step after another leading me to where I am today. The journey has not been necessarily just a physical one, slowly working my way toward one goal after another. It has also been an emotional and spiritual one, linking both my inner and outer worlds.

As you begin to read this book, you will soon discover that nurse practitioners work in a wide variety of settings and come from a diverse array of backgrounds. It is my belief that the rich diversity of experiences that nurse practitioners share makes up the collective awesomeness of the profession. Aside from the wealth of information within the text on how exactly to become a nurse practitioner, I've also included some of my own personal experiences and those of other nurse practitioners, as I hope that these tales will be helpful to you. Maybe you will find a common thread among our lives, and maybe you won't. Regardless of our similarities or differences, I hope that our stories help to guide and inspire you on your path to becoming a nurse practitioner.

It is my sincerest wish that you enjoy reading this book as much as I enjoyed researching and writing it. If some of the information within these pages does not resonate with you, no worries; take what works and leave the rest. I realize that we all learn differently and no one's life path is like another. Remember, the journey IS the destination. Buckle up and enjoy the ride!

My Story

I myself am made entirely of flaws, stitched together with good intentions.
—Augusten Burroughs

After graduating with a bachelor's degree from the University of Arizona, I joined the Peace Corps and spent two years volunteering in Cameroon, a geographically and ethnically diverse country located in Central Africa. I'd always wanted to be a Peace Corps Volunteer as far back as I can remember. When I was in high school I'd find myself on the internet looking at photos of volunteers in rural villages that were posted on their website. I'd often dream that one day it would be me and continued to nurse this dream throughout my high school and college years. Peace Corps service actually runs in my blood as my aunt was also a Peace Corps Volunteer who served in South America. She used to entertain me with her tales about rural life as a volunteer, and I was fascinated by her experiences.

Despite being a lifelong fan of the Peace Corps, when it was time to actually apply I almost didn't do it. Right before I graduated from college I had decided I would not apply as I was in a long-distance relationship and did not want things to end. However, a chance encounter on Halloween with my roommate's friend who was dressed as a bee changed everything. She was also a former Peace Corps Volunteer who served in Latin America. She made it clear to me that if I didn't go now, I'd probably never go. I took those words to heart and started my application that very night.

Less than a year later my lifelong dream of joining the Peace Corps finally turned into a reality. After a pre-departure orientation stateside, I and a group of both health and agriculture volunteers were flown to Cameroon via Paris. I arrived in Central Africa at the ripe old age of 21 with no idea of what I was getting myself into. I spent the first three months in Africa sweating to death in a rural village in Northern Cameroon while undergoing training with my fellow volunteers. I lived with a homestay family who had no electricity or running water, and food was cooked over an open fire. It was an amazing experience yet incredibly challenging as I struggled to learn French and assimilate into an entirely new culture, while also missing modern-day luxuries. After I finished training, I spent the next two years in a mountainous remote village near the Nigerian border where I would be serving as a health and community development volunteer.

During my time in Cameroon I bounced from hospital to clinic and even to the local jail teaching people and patients about health-related topics, working with community groups, planting trees—, just trying to make a small dent in the world. From kids' camps to pick-up soccer games, I was very involved with village life. I really loved the two years that I spent in Cameroon and even returned while in NP school where I did a clinical rotation at the local hospital. I still communicate often with the friends and acquaintances I made while I was a volunteer.

Despite my numerous exciting adventures, I also witnessed an incredible amount of poverty and human suffering, especially in the hospital setting. Patients slept on beds without mattresses or slept on mats on the floor while their relatives constantly swatted flies away from their lifeless faces. HIV, tuberculosis, and malaria were rampant and for many people, one of these diseases could mean a death sentence. As the hospital had no kitchen, if patients' families did not bring them food on a daily basis, then the patient would not eat. This is a concept that still haunts me today as I believe good nutrition is absolutely vital to the healing process.

As a volunteer I worked closely with a local doctor who would later become one of my closest friends and who also inspired me to work in the health field. My doctor friend worked tirelessly taking care of patients while battling with faulty (if any) electricity, rampant tropical diseases, language barriers (there are over 200 languages spoken in Cameroon!) and a lack of medicine and resources. Even though I left Cameroon years ago, my doctor friend continues to provide me with inspiration to be a better healthcare professional. I'm still amazed at his courage and dedication to the people of Cameroon.

For some reason while I was a Peace Corps Volunteer these health experiences didn't point me to a healthcare career but spurred me to want to become a human rights lawyer. Was it because I thought that tackling public health was too daunting? Did I prefer to stay on the policy side of things to make change on a greater level? Who knows, but to this day I still marvel at how terrible a lawyer I would have been (many of my friends and family also agree with this!).

Nevertheless, while still serving as a volunteer in Cameroon I tried very hard to get into law school. I researched admissions criteria during my weekly (or monthly) internet visits, consulted with friends and family on schools, and tried to learn as much as I could about the process to become a lawyer. I even studied for the law school admission test (LSAT) at night by oil lantern when my electricity was cut off. You would have thought that the second degree burn I received when my lantern tipped over and almost lit my mosquito net on fire would have been a sign that I was on the wrong path, but alas it was not.

I scheduled myself to take the LSAT in Cameroon (who does that?!) which was a big hassle and quite expensive to arrange. It took me two days to get to the capital city just to sit for the exam! From all the struggling I did just to set up and prepare for the exam, it wasn't a huge shocker that I didn't do very well once test day arrived. There were several other volunteers who also took the test with me and who eventually went on to law school. Although determined as ever to succeed on a path I clearly wasn't supposed to be on, I continued to pursue this misguided dream of becoming a human rights lawyer.

After my Peace Corps service was completed and I returned to the United States, I was still incredibly driven to go to law school. I spent several thousand dollars on an LSAT preparation course and dedicated three months to studying for the test. In hindsight, this money would have been much better spent on a new wardrobe and makeover from my post-African travels (and lack of style). But stubborn as ever I continued forward, ignoring all the signs that clearly indicated I wasn't meant to be a lawyer.

While enrolled in the LSAT study course, which took up a lot of my time, I began to notice that something just didn't feel right. I kept receiving poor scores on the LSAT practice tests, and even though I knew that the test didn't test my intelligence, I felt incredibly inept. I was very frustrated that all of my effort was taking me exactly nowhere. It was as if I was trying to fight the current of life and only being met with resistance.

A few weeks before I was going to take the test for a second time I had an epiphany. This happened during a brief, albeit life-changing conversation, with a psychic whom I met at a bar in West Seattle (this may make me lose credibility to a few readers but hey, it's the truth and needs to be told). Needless to say, that conversation caused me to do some serious soul-searching into my current predicament. After a visit to a local naturopathic medicine school where I had an extraordinarily powerful realization in their chapel, I decided not to take the LSAT. I am forever grateful to that woman, whoever she is, for forever altering my life's course and being the catalyst for me to take my first steps toward becoming a nurse practitioner. I've found that although I am incredibly stubborn and often struggle against my life's path, the universe always manages to get my attention (usually through another person) and lovingly guides me back to where I need to be.

The week after I decided not to take the non-refundable LSAT exam (yet again, more wasted money, but cheaper than failing out of law school!) I enrolled in my first-ever college-level science course at the local community college (I took geology as an undergraduate but don't really think that counts in this context). This class was the first of the following ten courses or so that I would take over the next two years prior to even applying to a nurse practitioner program.

While I was completing my prerequisite courses, things didn't get much easier for me. I'd wake up at five o'clock in the morning to study for a few hours and then I'd head to my part-time job at a local non-profit. After work, I'd drive to the community college where I'd take my classes, which were usually later in the day or at night. Some days I was so exhausted I would sleep in my car in between classes, trying to catch up on some much-needed sleep.

It was during one of these many courses and after deciding that the nurse practitioner route was the one for me (I had also strongly considered both medical school and naturopathic medicine school) that I had a conversation with a classmate regarding our future careers. I didn't particularly like this student as I thought she was arrogant and condescending. However, during the course of our conversation she said she was applying to Columbia University's family nurse practitioner (FNP) program. I didn't even know Columbia had any NP programs but I was interested so I applied. Months later and to my surprise, I was accepted into the FNP program at Columbia University School of Nursing. Once again Lady Fate had intervened and my life's course was steered in the right direction.

As you can see from my story, so many things had to happen (or not happen) in order for me to become a nurse practitioner. The path hasn't necessarily been an easy one; it's been downright challenging—often producing extreme highs and lows. However, looking back on the journey, I wouldn't change it for the world.

· 1 ·

DEFINING THE NURSE PRACTITIONER

Let me dedicate my life today to the care of those who come my way. Let me touch each one with a healing hand and the gentle art for which I stand. And then tonight when the day is done, let me rest in peace if I've helped just one.

—Unknown

For more than half a century, nurse practitioners have been helping to shape primary care and the overall health of this nation. From outpatient clinics to working in the intensive care unit (ICU), NPs can be found in virtually every corner of health care. Not only do nurse practitioners diagnose and manage patients in a wide variety of settings, but they also have also been in the forefront of shaping policy for the profession and advocating for change in the best interests of their patients.

To understand exactly what a nurse practitioner is and what the role entails, we need to start by understanding just how the profession started and how it has evolved since its inception. Like many other professions that have arrived where they are today, nurse practitioners have had to struggle every step of the way—often fighting multiple battles at a time. Since the birth of the profession was just a little over fifty years ago, a lot has happened from the time that nurse practitioners came into the workforce to the status that they hold today.

History of the Nurse Practitioner

During the 1960s, there were community health nurses that were incredibly independent, especially those in rural and underserved communities. It's important to note that people who live in medically underserved communities often lack access to healthcare providers and basic medical services, which in turn negatively affects their health. Unfortunately, this was the case back then and still holds true today. To reach those in need, these community health nurses often traveled to visit their patients regardless of where they lived, and were the eyes and ears of the supervising physician with whom they worked in close collaboration. Often the patients they treated had complex medical needs that they did not have the knowledge or the expertise to manage. Physicians began to mentor these nurses and collaborate with them in order to best serve their patients (O'Brien, 2003).

In 1965, both Medicare and Medicaid were created to provide medical services for low-income children and women, the elderly, and those who had disabilities. As a whole new population of people were suddenly insured, primary care facilities were overwhelmed by the influx of new patients. In addition to this large surge of patients, there was also a primary care physician shortage (which is still true today) as many primary care physicians had transitioned into specialty practice. With more and more insured patients needing medical care and physicians already taxed by the physician shortage, nurses were in the perfect position to fill the gap for those in need. Thus, a new career was born: the nurse practitioner (O'Brien, 2003).

Pioneered by nurse leader Dr. Loretta Ford and pediatrician Dr. Henry Silver, the first nurse practitioner program was started in 1965 at the University of Colorado Health Sciences Center (Historical Timeline, 2017; O'Brien, 2003). The nurses enrolled in this program were taught how to perform a more comprehensive physical exam, assess the patient, and manage them based on their findings. The curriculum focused on promoting health and preventing disease in children and the family. This program, which changed the role of a nurse to that of a healthcare provider, was the catalyst for the nurse practitioner movement. Once this program was established, this newly formed career took off running.

Although nurse practitioners were originally trained to work in the community health sector, this soon transitioned to them working in the primary care arena, eventually becoming primary care providers (PCPs). By 1973, just eight years after the inception of the first nurse practitioner program, there were sixty-five established nurse practitioner programs around the country with more being created each year (Historical Timeline, 2017).

As nurse practitioners made headway with political and legislative movements, they also faced enormous resistance. The rise in nurse practitioner status from nurse to clinician created significant backlash among other healthcare professionals, coming from both physicians and nurses alike. Nursing professionals felt that nurses who took on this new role as a nurse practitioner were no longer adhering to the traditional nursing model. Concomitantly physicians criticized NPs because they did not have the training or the education to function in this newly defined role (O'Brien, 2003). Nevertheless, these brave nurses and nurse practitioners continued to charge ahead, not letting this fierce opposition stop them. Regardless of the criticism from other healthcare professions, nurse practitioners have proven over and over again that they provide excellent patient care.

As history tends to repeat itself, with the implementation of the 2010 Affordable Care Act millions of newly insured patients sought out healthcare services similar to the implementation of Medicaid and Medicare in the 1960s. With this new flood of patients, NPs were yet again called to fill the void to provide patient care to those who needed it most. Today nurse practitioners still face opposition from others hoping to quiet their strong voice. Legislative bodies continue to prevent nurse practitioners from working to the full extent of their training. Some state regulations prevent nurse practitioners from providing certain services to their patients, while in other states they are allowed to do so. These old-fashioned regulations not only limit the nurse practitioner, but these laws trickle down and affect the patient as well.

Despite outdated laws, today more than ever there is reason to be optimistic about the future of the NP profession. State laws continue to evolve removing old jargon and barriers, and more nurse practitioners are now able to practice within the full breadth of their training. Changes in certain state legislations have also allowed nurse practitioners to manage their patients autonomously by removing physician collaboration requirements. It's a win-win situation for both patients and NPs! Although there are still many states that continue to impose restrictions on nurse practitioners, today many more NPs are enjoying increased autonomy and the ability to practice with fewer restrictions than they previously had. This is due to the courage and perseverance of earlier NPs.

These days it is an exciting time to be a nurse practitioner. We are able to continue to be the voice for the patients we serve and make changes that help to better the health of the nation. I'm very excited for the day when all nurse practitioners nationwide will be able to practice to the full extent of their training without limitations. As restrictions continue to fall by the wayside, that day may be coming sooner rather than later.

The Nurse Practitioner Role

Nurses have come a long way in a few short decades. In the past our attention focused on physical, mental and emotional healing. Now we talk of healing your life, healing the environment and healing the planet.

—Lynn Keegan

It's a beautiful thing when career and passion come together.

—Unknown

Now that you understand a bit more about the history of the nurse practitioner profession, let's shift gears to touch base on the *role* of a nurse practitioner. Prior to becoming an NP this caused some confusion on my part as I wasn't exactly sure about what the role and function of an NP entailed. Furthermore, many of my patients are often confused about my role and title as well. They think that I'm either a nurse or a doctor, not realizing there's a large middle ground.

I'm actually quite surprised when a patient is familiar with the term "nurse practitioner" and truly understands the function of a nurse practitioner. When you realize that your patient has been to an NP before you may also find out they chose to come to you because you are a nurse practitioner! They often have great things to say about their previous experience with a nurse practitioner, thus leading them into your care. One of my patients came to me after requesting at the front desk to not have a "white male doctor." When she showed up in my exam room and told me the story we laughed at how far I am from this.

Similar to the confusion that I've experienced, throughout your career as a nurse practitioner you will most likely meet many people who are confused about your role in the clinical setting. People may wonder how a nurse practitioner differs from other health professionals such as physicians and physician assistants. Your friends and family may also have quite a bit of confusion about nurse practitioners. For example, one of my good friends continues to call me a nurse despite my having told him 1000 times that I'm a *nurse practitioner*. He just doesn't understand that there is a huge difference between these two healthcare professions! You may even be confused yourself about what an NP is and are looking for more clarity as to what the career entails. Therefore, I think it's best to clarify what exactly is and what isn't a nurse practitioner.

To clear up any confusion I've included several frequently asked questions that may come up when you discuss your goal of becoming a nurse practitioner. I've found that it's best to have a couple of responses readily available regarding commonly asked questions to help explain what the role of an NP actually is. Additionally, if you are still unsure if the nurse practitioner profession is the right career choice for you, this section may help you decide if you want to pursue this field.

Nurse Practitioner Frequently Asked Questions

So, what exactly is a nurse practitioner?

This may seem like a simple question, but as I've alluded to above, you would be surprised how many people don't know what a nurse practitioner is. Not only are patients often confused about the role of the nurse practitioner, but so are other healthcare professionals. You will get asked this question often throughout your career so I thought it best to start off with the basics of the profession and build from there. Essentially, an NP is a registered nurse (RN) who has additional clinical training and education beyond that of an RN.

The nurse practitioner profession is under the umbrella term of advanced practice registered nurse (APRN). NPs are one of four advanced practice nursing professions with the others being certified nurse-midwives, certified registered nurse anesthetists, and clinical nurse specialists. To become an APRN you are required to have additional training beyond a registered nurse licensure, such as a master's and/or doctorate degree. The other three APRN specialties require training that is very different from NP training and each APRN specialty differs from one another. The one similarity among all four APRN specialties is that each is able to earn a terminal degree; the doctor of nursing practice (DNP) degree.

The definition of a nurse practitioner is a legal term and varies state by state. The wording used to describe a nurse practitioner is state dependent as well. As you progress through your training to become a nurse practitioner, you will start to understand more about what terms and language are used to describe NPs in your state. Once you familiarize yourself a bit more with the profession, the jargon surrounding your legal title and the scope of practice (more on this later in the text) for your state will sound less confusing.

Your legal title can also cause some confusion and is dependent on the state in which you practice. For example, in one state you may be legally called a nurse practitioner, yet in another state you are called an advanced practice registered nurse (or any other legal title that they give NPs). This caused me a lot of confusion when I moved from one state to another, as I went from being called a nurse practitioner to being called an advanced practice registered nurse.

What type of services do nurse practitioners provide?

Nurse practitioners perform many functions similar to physicians in the clinical setting, though they do not perform invasive surgery. The services that you will be providing depend upon your board certification, training, and facility where you work.

For example, if you are a board certified pediatric nurse practitioner you won't be treating elderly patients, and if you are a board certified adult nurse practitioner you won't be seeing neonates as patients. Additionally, the training you have will also determine the clinical services you provide. As a family nurse practitioner, I am legally allowed to perform procedures such as suturing and stapling. However, if I am not properly trained to do so then I should not perform these procedures. Where you work will also determine what other clinical skills you will be using. The clinical skills used by an NP in the ICU setting will be much different from that of an NP working in an outpatient primary care facility. Many of the clinical and procedural skills you will acquire may be taught in school, although they will also be learned at your job as well.

As you have probably begun to see, NPs provide a extensive array of services in a wide variety of settings. Below is a brief list of some of the services provided by nurse practitioners in the clinical setting to give you a better idea of what the profession entails. Keep in mind that this list is not all-inclusive and NPs perform many more additional services than those listed below. Nurse practitioners:

- Acquire a patient's medical history and perform a physical exam
- Diagnose and manage patients

- Screen patients for diseases and recommend the most appropriate screening tests
- Educate patients on their health and provide anticipatory guidance
- Write prescriptions for medications, vaccinations, durable medical equipment, etc.
- Order lab tests and imaging and interpret the results
- Refer to specialty care
- Deliver prenatal care and provide services for family planning
- Perform well child examinations including immunizing pediatric patients per guidelines
- Perform women's health gynecological exam
- Perform procedures
- Manage chronic illnesses

(Buppert, 2008). Remember, this is just a brief list of what NPs do in clinical practice. As you will see later on in the text, nurse practitioners can be found working in practically any healthcare setting while performing a number of different functions.

Do nurse practitioners provide patient education?

Yes! At the core of the nurse practitioner profession is a large education component. In my work as a nurse practitioner I am continually educating and counseling my patients on healthier living and better lifestyles. I know that many of my NP colleagues also provide extensive patient education. Additionally, NPs tend to look at their patients holistically, treating the entire patient as a whole, and not just treating the disease. This may include counseling on healthy eating habits, educating a patient on medication side effects, exercise recommendations, stress reduction techniques, and suggestions on living a healthier lifestyle.

What do the terms mid-level practitioner and physician extender mean?

Nurse practitioners have also been referred to as "mid-level practitioners" and "physician extenders," two terms that I and many of my colleagues do not necessarily care for. Nurse practitioners are a profession unto themselves and are not mid-level in anything they do. Although NPs have less training than physicians, we still provide excellent patient care. The term "mid-level practitioner" is a legal term used by the Drug Enforcement Administration (DEA).

This term identifies a subset of healthcare providers as a way to monitor controlled-substance prescriptions (Bishop, 2012).

Additionally, the term "physician extender" is not accurate either. Nurse practitioners are not extensions of physicians; they are their colleagues. Nurse practitioners work under their own license and in many states do not need any sort of collaborative physician agreement to practice. Nurse practitioners however do often work together in collaborative relationships with physicians (professionally not legally) as they realize that working together with other medical disciplines is best for their patients. If an NP is unable to meet the needs of a patient, then they may refer to other specialties, sometimes, but not always, referring to physicians. Concomitantly, NPs also treat patients that our physician colleagues refer to us!

To see what the American Association of Nurse Practitioners (AANP) feels about these terms "mid-level provider" and "physician extender" visit their website at www.aanp.org/images/documents/publications/useofterms.pdf

What type of education does a nurse practitioner have?

Prior to the inception of the master's degree requirement for nurse practitioners, many nurses in NP school were enrolled in certificate programs that have since been replaced with the master's level programs, doctoral level programs, and post-master's certificate programs. Although there are NPs who still practice with a certificate, over 95% of practicing nurse practitioners have a graduate level degree (NP Fact Sheet, 2017).

Even though the large majority of nurse practitioners are currently practicing at the master's level, the AANP had decided to transition nurse practitioners from a master's prepared profession to a doctorally prepared profession by 2015. So, what does this mean exactly? NPs that have been practicing under a certificate or master's degree will be grandfathered in without having to receive their doctorate in order to continue practicing. However, future NPs will be required to obtain their doctorate.

This initiative also affects nurse practitioner programs as graduate schools have started to eliminate the master's portion and go straight to the Doctor of Nursing Practice degree—more commonly known as the DNP. Although this mandate has not yet been fully implemented, more and more NPs are receiving their DNP. As many other health professions are already prepared at the doctoral level, nurse practitioners have the opportunity to have a terminal degree as well.

What is the difference between a DNP and PhD in nursing?

Both the DNP (Doctor of Nursing Practice) and PhD (Doctor of Philosophy) are doctorate level nursing degrees. Essentially, the DNP degree is a clinically-based degree while the PhD is a research-based degree. Graduates of either degree can work as a nurse practitioner once they have completed their NP studies and are certified in their specialty. The majority of NPs with a doctorate degree hold the DNP degree.

Do nurse practitioners write prescriptions?

Heck yeah, we do! There will be more on nurse practitioner prescribing later on in the text.

What is the difference between a nurse practitioner and a registered nurse?

This is another common question you will get once you start your NP program and/or job. People may still refer to you as a nurse even while working as a nurse practitioner as there is still a lot of confusion among the general public between these two healthcare roles.

The education, training, and what each profession is legally allowed to do is much different between a registered nurse and a nurse practitioner. As stated earlier, a nurse practitioner is an advanced practice registered nurse with a bachelor of science in nursing and either a master's and/or doctorate degree in nursing. A registered nurse has either an associate's degree or bachelor's degree in nursing.

As far as training goes, RNs are trained to be nurses, while NPs are trained to be healthcare providers. NPs have much more autonomy and additional clinical training than an RN. Although many times NPs and RNs work together as colleagues in similar settings, the role of an RN and an NP differs greatly.

Legally RNs are not allowed to perform many of the functions that an NP can perform. Unlike RNs, NPs can write prescriptions, refer to other specialties, be considered primary care providers, and perform certain medical procedures that nurses are not allowed to perform. It is important to keep in mind that you must first be a registered nurse prior to becoming a nurse practitioner. Legally, if your RN license is expired or suspended in the state in which you are licensed, then you cannot work as a nurse practitioner in that state.

If I am a nurse practitioner can I still work as a nurse?

Yes! I've worked as an RN while I've been an NP and many of my friends do as well. It's a great way to supplement your income and also learn additional skills at each position you hold. That's part of the beauty of this profession; there is a lot of flexibility, growth, and diversity.

What is the difference between a nurse practitioner and a physician assistant (PA)?

Nurse practitioners and physician assistants perform many similar tasks on the job. Both professions diagnose and treat patients, prescribe medications, and work in a variety of clinical areas. Similar to NPs, PAs can also specialize in various areas of medicine; however, they tend to work more in surgical settings than NPs do. The main difference between PAs and NPs is the training and licensure. Physician assistants follow the medical model similar to physicians, sometimes taking science courses concomitantly with medical students. They have shorter training than physicians and, unlike NPs, do not have to be registered nurses before entering their field.

As far as licensure goes both professions carry their own licenses; however, PAs must always be supervised or have a collaborative agreement with a licensed physician and cannot practice without these arrangements. The level of supervision depends on the state—some states require the physician to be in the building while other states may only require the physician to be available by phone. Nurse practitioners work independently in many states, and depending on the state may not need any sort of physician collaboration in order to practice. As you can see NPs hold more autonomy than PAs; however, this is autonomy in a legal sense as both professions see patients on their own, often doing so without any physician intervention.

NPs and PAs can also be found working side by side in the clinical setting. You'll often see job advertisements looking for an NP/PA to fill the position. We perform a lot of the same functions and consult each other when needed. I worked with a very knowledgeable and seasoned PA who was a great mentor and a great PA. He taught me a lot, and on occasion would come to me with questions regarding things he wasn't certain about as well. I enjoyed working with him and both of our skill sets complemented each other.

I've asked people who are attending PA school or are deciding to become a PA instead of an NP what made them decide PA over NP. Many told me it was because they didn't want to become a nurse. If you're in a similar situation where you want to go into the medical field and become a medical provider but don't want to be a physician or a nurse practitioner, then becoming a PA may be suitable for you and I suggest you look more into this profession. Not that I'm trying to sway anyone from becoming an NP, but this book is also designed to help you decide if you don't want to become an NP.

What is the difference between a nurse practitioner and a physician?

I don't know how many times I've been asked the question, "So why didn't you just become a doctor?" One of my RN colleagues who also wants to be an NP even asked me this question! It's as if the person asking this question has little to no regard for the massive amounts of time and money I've invested into getting to where I am today, a board-certified family nurse practitioner with a doctorate degree. Instead of getting annoyed or angry, I've chosen to put on a smile and educate whomever I'm speaking to about the role of a nurse practitioner and why I chose this profession instead of going to medical school. Not to say that this question doesn't sometimes get under my skin because it often does. However, educating people and patients about the role of a nurse practitioner is a crucial part of advocating for our profession.

Essentially nurse practitioners do many of the same things that physicians do in a clinical setting (though as stated previously NPs do not perform invasive surgery). The difference between an NP and a physician is in education, definition of the profession, and scope of practice (Buppert, 2008). The training for physicians is much longer and more extensive than the training to be a nurse practitioner. We also belong to different board certifying organizations and have different requirements for obtaining and maintaining our licenses.

However, clinically we are often working side by side seeing many of the same patients. Oftentimes if you are in a clinical setting you may not be able to tell who is who by looking at the provider. Where I've worked I see the same patients as the physicians and we perform the exact same job functions. At other locations this may be different, as it depends on where you work and also the billing structure of your organization.

Do nurse practitioners offer quality patient care?

Yes, and there are numerous studies to prove it! Nevertheless, this answer obviously depends on the individual who is treating the patient. There will always be healthcare providers who provide substandard care, whether they are a nurse practitioner or part of another healthcare profession. However, studies have shown that, as a whole, nurse practitioners produce similar outcomes to physicians in the primary care setting. Nurse practitioners consistently perform well with both patient satisfaction and the medical management of disease.

One such study performed by Swan, Ferguson, Chang, Larson, and Smaldone (2015) is a systematic review of the quality of care provided by advanced practice nurses (APNs) in the primary care setting. The study found that APNs performed similar to physicians on certain measures, and better than physicians on other measures. Another study performed by Stanik-Hutt et al. (2013) found similar results with evidence showing that "NPs provide high quality, safe, and effective patient care."

These are just two of the many studies that have been carried out demonstrating just how safe and effective nurse practitioner managed care is. I encourage you to continue doing your research into outcomes of nurse practitioner care because the research is inspiring to read and also useful when people have questions about the safety and efficacy of the NP profession.

Do nurse practitioners specialize in a particular area?

Yes, as an NP you will have a primary specialty area under which you are licensed. You also have the option to subspecialize, which may mean taking additional courses in that subspecialty area. There will be more on sub-specialization later on in the text. Below is a list of primary areas in which nurse practitioners can specialize.

- Pediatric nurse practitioner (primary care and acute care)
- Adult gerontology nurse practitioner (primary care and acute care)
- Family nurse practitioner
- Psychiatric and mental health nurse practitioner
- Women's health nurse practitioner
- Neonatal nurse practitioner

Now that I understand what a nurse practitioner is, how do I know if I want to become a nurse practitioner?

Unfortunately, this question must come from within and I can only help guide you on your journey to making that decision. Deciding if you really truly want to be a nurse practitioner is a big decision. Years of preparation and dedication go into becoming a nurse practitioner, and this decision shouldn't be taken lightly. This question requires a bit of soul-searching, and if you are not sure becoming a nurse practitioner is what you want to do, I suggest you continue reading this book as well as conduct your own research as this may better assist you with your decision.

If you like helping people and enjoy the challenges of medicine, then becoming a nurse practitioner may be your calling. However, if you're not yet ready to take the plunge and need a little more information on what the job is actually like, then I suggest you try and shadow an NP in the clinical setting. This will allow you to get a feel for what daily life can be like working as an NP. Granted each NP functions differently and no two health settings are the same; however, at least you will get some sort of idea of what NPs do and how they interact with their patients. You can also reach out to your local NP organization to speak with an NP about the profession. Additionally, if you have any family or friends who are NPs, talk to them about their job. NPs tend to be helpful and I'll bet you will find several who would be happy to help you out.

On the next page I've created Table 1.1 for you to jot down some of the reasons why you may or may not like to pursue this field. I find that writing things down and reflecting on them often helps make an important decision a little less difficult. Feel free to list as many things in each column such as cost of education or quality of life. Referencing this chart throughout this book and adding to it also may help you make this decision.

Table 1.1. Reasons to pursue a career as an NP versus reasons not to pursue a career as an NP.

Reasons to pursue a career as a Nurse Practitioner	Reasons NOT to pursue a career as a Nurse Practitioner

Source: Author.

Nurse Practitioner Scope of Practice and State Practice Environments

I hope that the previous section provided you with a bit more clarity on exactly what is and what isn't a nurse practitioner. However, understanding the role and function of a nurse practitioner is not the entirety of the profession. We now must look at what a nurse practitioner is legally allowed to do by understanding the following terms: scope of practice and state practice environments.

Scope of Practice

As a nurse practitioner, you will most likely hear the term "scope of practice," and it is an important concept that should be understood. I first heard this phrase as a nursing student, and it was often discussed throughout my NP curriculum. Essentially scope of practice means what a nurse practitioner can legally do underneath his or her professional licensure and certification. In the United States, nurse practitioner scope of practice is determined at the state level by the state nursing regulatory body, usually the state board of nursing. Each state has its own rules and regulations that determine the scope of practice for the NP, with some states allowing NPs much more autonomy than others. The American Association of Nurse Practitioners (AANP) defines scope of practice in the professional role as:

> Nurse practitioners (NPs) are licensed, independent practitioners who practice in ambulatory, acute and long-term care as primary and/or specialty care providers. Nurse practitioners assess, diagnose, treat, and manage acute episodic and chronic illnesses. NPs are experts in health promotion and disease prevention. They order, conduct, supervise, and interpret diagnostic and laboratory tests, prescribe pharmacological agents and non-pharmacologic therapies, as well as teach and counsel patients, among other services.

> As licensed, independent clinicians, NPs practice autonomously and in coordination with health care professionals and other individuals. They may serve as health care researchers, interdisciplinary consultants, and patient advocates. NPs provide a wide-range of health care services to individuals, families, groups, and communities. (Scope of Practice for Nurse Practitioners, n.d.)

State Practice Environments

Another phrase you may come across is state practice environment. This is a term used to discuss how much autonomy an NP has at the state level. There are three types of state practice environments under which the NP practices: full practice environment (also referred to as full practice authority), reduced practice environment, and restricted practice environment. A full practice environment is the most autonomous and a restricted practice environment is the most restrictive. For example, some states require that NPs have a collaborative relationship with a physician, while others do not. Additionally, in some states NPs are allowed to sign death certificates, but in others they may not. You get the picture; how much autonomy an NP is granted depends on the state in which they practice.

The American Association of Nurse Practitioners (AANP) is a great resource with even more information regarding state practice environments. This can be found at www.aanp.org/legislation-regulation/state-legislation/state-practice-environment.

This website is an excellent way to understand which states have stricter regulations regarding NP practice. It's interesting to see how NP state practice environments are regionally grouped. The western part of the country generally allows NPs to have the most autonomy with more full practice states, and the south is the most restrictive with more restricted practice states. It's also interesting to note that one state could have full practice authority but share a state border with a state where NPs have a restricted practice. Full practice authority for all nurse practitioners is the model recommended by both the National Council of State Boards of Nursing as well as the Institute of Medicine (Committee on the Robert Wood Johnson Foundation Initiative on the Future of Nursing, at the Institute of Medicine, 2011).

Nurse practitioner scope of practice and state practice environments may also help you determine the state in which you want to live. As a nurse practitioner working in a full practice state, I think it would be very challenging to move to a restricted practice state as I am used to full autonomy underneath my licensure. Also, if I move to a reduced or restricted practice state, I have to be cognizant of what I can legally do as an NP. This is definitely something to keep in mind if you receive your training in one state, and then move to another one after graduation. Some NPs find restricted practice cumbersome, while for others it's more regulatory in nature and does not affect their day to day practice.

The conversation regarding scope of practice barriers and state practice environment regulations have caused a lot of controversy as nurse practitioners continuously advocate for their rights and for full practice authority. The goal is for all nurse practitioners to be autonomous healthcare providers who do not need any sort of physician collaboration or oversight. As the nurse practitioner profession continues to evolve, my hope is that nurse practitioners will have full practice authority in all fifty states in the near future. With the growing need for more healthcare providers, and more and more patients getting insurance, this may occur sooner rather than later.

Advanced Practice Registered Nurse Regulatory Model

Similar to other health care professions, nurse practitioners must be regulated. The licensure, accreditation, certification and education (LACE) of nurse practitioners and other advanced practice registered nurses (APRNs) such as certified nurse-midwives, clinical nurse specialists, and certified registered nurse anesthetists is governed by several different professional organizations. For example, the organization that accredits your nurse practitioner program is different from the organization which oversees your state license. According to *The Future of Nursing: Leading Change, Advancing Health* the terms under LACE are defined as:

> Licensure is the granting of authority to practice. Accreditation is the formal review and approval by a recognized agency of educational degree or certification programs in nursing or nursing-related programs. Certification is the formal recognition of the knowledge, skills, and experience demonstrated by the achievement of standards identified by the profession. Education is the formal preparation of APRNs in graduate degree-granting or post-graduate certificate programs. (Committee on the Robert Wood Johnson Foundation Initiative on the Future of Nursing, at the Institute of Medicine, 2011)

Although the wording and professional jargon may seem a bit confusing, don't worry too much about these terms and what they mean. I just wanted to mention them so that you have some understanding about how the profession is regulated and structured. Later on in the text, there will be more information on obtaining the license and certification you will need in order to work as a nurse practitioner.

Institute of Medicine Report

In 2010 the Institute of Medicine (IOM) and the Robert Wood Johnson Foundation highlighted the need for nurse practitioners to practice to the full scope and breadth of their knowledge. Although this report emphasized barriers that nurses of all levels face, nurse practitioner barriers to practice was the first recommendation that the report addressed, and the IOM advocated for change at multiple levels. This report was a big win for nurse practitioners as the IOM is an independent institution that is not affiliated with nursing. Below is a brief summary of the eight recommendations that the Institute of Medicine published for nurses, nurse practitioners, and the APRN profession (Committee on the Robert Wood Johnson Foundation Initiative on the Future of Nursing, at the Institute of Medicine, 2011).

(1) "Remove scope-of-practice barriers" for advanced practice registered nurses.
(2) "Expand opportunities for nurses to lead and diffuse collaborative improvement efforts."
(3) "Implement nurse residency programs."
(4) "Increase the proportion of nurses with a baccalaureate degree to 80 percent by 2020."
(5) "Double the number of nurses with a doctorate by 2020."
(6) "Ensure that nurses engage in lifelong learning."
(7) "Prepare and enable nurses to lead change to advance health."
(8) "Build an infrastructure for the collection and analysis of interprofessional health care workforce data."

Although these recommendations were put forth in 2010, due to policy and legislature the recommendations have not yet been fully implemented. However, if the future of the nurse practitioner profession is anything like the past, we will continue to fight outdated laws to ensure we are granted the rights that we have earned.

Prescriptive Authority

Fortunately, the one thing that nurse practitioners in all 50 states (including Washington, D.C.) do hold in common is that NPs have prescriptive authority (NP Fact Sheet, 2017). This means nurse practitioners can write prescriptions including prescribing controlled substances once they have their federal DEA number. In addition to a DEA number, some states also require an additional license to prescribe controlled substances. The state under which an NP is licensed will determine what controlled substances a nurse practitioner can and cannot prescribe.

Prescriptive authority does not just include pharmacologic therapies but also includes durable medical equipment and other medical supplies. On average, a full-time nurse practitioner writes around 23 prescriptions per day (NP Fact Sheet, 2017). Depending on the state where you live (do you see a trend here?) you may get your prescriptive authority when you get your NP license, or you may have to apply for it separately. You may have to take additional pharmacology continuing education courses to maintain your prescriptive authority; it depends on your state laws. If you have any questions about the prescriptive authority laws or application process, make sure you clarify them with the state board of nursing.

Advanced Practice Registered Nurse Terms

During your journey to become an NP, you will most likely come across a plethora of terms pertaining to the nurse practitioner profession. Becoming a nurse practitioner is challenging enough without having to learn all the different acronyms and language that comes along with it! For this reason, I created the list below to help clarify any confusion. As you will see, nurse practitioners can be called by several names and acronyms yet do the exact same job. Some of the terms below are more common than others, and some mean the same thing, just stated differently. It is important to remember that this is not a complete list of all nurse practitioner terms, and if you come across an NP term aside from those listed below, please feel free to include it. Additionally, this list also includes other acronyms, some of which are not nurse practitioners but are included under the umbrella term of advanced practice registered nurse.

- ACNP Acute Care Nurse Practitioner
- ACPNP Acute Care Pediatric Nurse Practitioner
- AGNP Adult Gerontology Nurse Practitioner
- AGACNP Adult Gerontology Acute Care Nurse Practitioner
- AGPCNP Adult Gerontology Primary Care Nurse Practitioner
- ANP Adult Nurse Practitioner

- ANP Advanced Nurse Practitioner
- AOCNP Advanced Oncology Certified Nurse Practitioner
- APN Advanced Practice Nurse
- APNP Advanced Practice Nurse Prescriber
- APRN Advanced Practice Registered Nurse
- ARNP Advanced Registered Nurse Practitioner
- BC Board Certified
- C Certified
- CNM Certified Nurse-Midwife
- CNP Certified Nurse Practitioner
- CRNA Certified Registered Nurse Anesthetist
- CRNP Certified Registered Nurse Practitioner
- CNS Clinical Nurse Specialist
- DCNP Dermatology Certified Nurse Practitioner
- DNP Doctor of Nursing Practice
- ENP Emergency Nurse Practitioner
- FNP Family Nurse Practitioner
- GNP Gerontological Nurse Practitioner
- NNP Neonatal Nurse Practitioner
- NP Nurse Practitioner
- ONP-C Certified Orthopedic Nurse Practitioner
- PMHNP Psychiatric-Mental Health Nurse Practitioner
- PNP Pediatric Nurse Practitioner
- PNP-AC Pediatric Nurse Practitioner, Acute Care
- PNP-PC Pediatric Nurse Practitioner, Primary Care
- RNP Registered Nurse Practitioner
- SNP School Nurse Practitioner
- WHNP Women's Health Nurse Practitioner

Nurse Practitioners in the Workforce

Now that the basics of the nurse practitioner profession have been spelled out, let's look at NPs in the workforce. As of 2017, there are over 234,000 practicing licensed nurse practitioners in the United States (NP Fact Sheet, 2017). This number continues to grow as more and more nurses and other professionals decide to enroll in nurse practitioner programs. This number is even more incredible if you consider the fact that a little over 50 years ago, there were no nurse practitioners at all!

If you are already familiar with the profession you may have some sort of idea where nurse practitioners can be found working. However, if you have no idea where nurse practitioners work, get ready to be impressed as we are everywhere! The rest of this chapter is dedicated to highlighting the incredible diversity of job options that are available to nurse practitioners.

Where Do Nurse Practitioners Work?

One of the great things about working as a nurse practitioner is having the ability to choose between a wide variety of places and specialties in which to work. Just a quick browse on the internet for nurse practitioner jobs will show just how in demand this profession is, and all the various locations where nurse practitioners can be found. Although the majority of nurse practitioners are certified in primary care (almost 90%; NP Fact Sheet, 2017), there are a multitude of other healthcare settings besides a primary care facility where NPs are employed.

Another great thing about being a nurse practitioner is that you can also switch clinical settings based on your interest. A nurse practitioner who works in cardiology can change jobs to work in endocrinology or vice versa without having to receive additional formal training (although there will be on-the-job training) or being required to complete an additional exam. Obviously if you are board certified to see only adults you cannot change jobs to work in pediatrics without additional certification; however, that's across the board. The amazing thing about this profession is that it is incredibly versatile and provides for an unbelievable amount of growth on both the personal and professional level.

Below is a list of some of the places where you may find yourself working as a nurse practitioner. Remember this list is not all-inclusive so if there is a specialty in which you want to work, chances are they may hire an NP.

- Acute care
- Addiction/Chemical Dependency
- Adolescent/Teen Clinic
- Allergy & Immunology
- Assisted Living Facility
- Bariatric Surgery
- Cardiology
- College/University Health Clinic

- Community Health Clinic
- Correctional Facility
- Dermatology
- Endocrinology
- Emergency Department
- Family Medicine
- Functional Medicine
- Gastroenterology
- General Surgery
- Geriatrics
- Health Department
- Hematology
- Hepatology
- Home Health. This can mean a variety of things, from providing house calls to patients to performing in-home physical exams and assessments for insurance companies.
- Homeless Shelter
- Hospital Inpatient Unit. Hospitalist care is also incredibly diverse giving NPs a wide variety of options within the inpatient hospital setting.
- Infectious Disease
- Intensive Care Unit (ICU)
- Medical Spa
- Mobile Health Unit. This is a clinic located in a van or bus that travels to different locations serving patients and providing medical and/or dental services. It is usually designed to serve rural and/or underserved communities.
- Military Base or Veterans Affairs Facility
- Multispecialty Practice
- Neonatology
- Nephrology
- Neurology
- Obstetrics and Gynecology
- Oncology
- Orthopedics
- Otolaryngology
- Pain Management
- Palliative Care

- Pediatrics
- Pediatric Specialty Practice
- Plastic Surgery
- Primary Care
- Private Practice
- Psychiatry/Mental Health Facility
- Pulmonology
- Rehabilitation Facility
- Retail-based Clinic such as the Minute Clinic located in CVS
- Rheumatology
- Rural Health
- School-based Clinic
- Skilled Nursing Facility
- Summer Camp
- Telemedicine
- Travel Medicine
- Tropical Medicine
- University Faculty/Teaching
- Urgent Care
- Urology
- Weight Loss Clinic
- Women's Health Clinic
- Wound Care

Nurse Practitioner Work Schedules

As you have just read, a wonderful thing about working as a nurse practitioner is that you have an incredible amount of flexibility and choice of where you want to work. Additionally, you may even have the choice to decide exactly how much you want to work. Just seeing the list above of where nurse practitioners can be employed should give you an idea of just how much work is out there for NPs. There are thousands of nurse practitioner jobs advertised on the internet with more and more being posted every day.

As stated above, as a nurse practitioner you may have flexibility on how much you want to work as well. If a job posts that they want someone to work five days a week, but you want Fridays off, you may be able to negotiate a four-day work week. Or if they post about a 40-hour work week schedule, and you don't want to work more than 35 hours, this may be negotiable too.

Additionally, potential employers may also work around your schedule. If you have a fixed day or time during the week that you cannot work, you may be able to work around your previous commitment. This is an added bonus if you already have another job and/or other obligation.

Depending on where you work, your hours may be fixed or they may be flexible. You may find yourself working four hours at a time or twelve hours at time; it depends on your facility's needs along with your personal preferences and availability. Aside from the typical 40-hour work week, there are nurse practitioners who opt to work a part-time per diem schedule. This means that they work as needed for their employer without the constraints of a fixed schedule. As a per diem employee you may not receive perks such as benefits and paid time off; however, per diem gives you freedom to dictate your own schedule, something that many NPs find very attractive. You could even combine both a fixed schedule with a per diem job if this suits your needs.

Many nurse practitioners also opt to work locum tenens jobs, which can be incredibly lucrative. Locum tenens, from the Latin phrase "holding one's place," in general means someone filling in for a temporary position. Locum tenens agencies often help fill company vacancies for short-term contract work if a permanent employee is out for a period of time. Locum tenens can also be used if a company predicts an influx of patients and needs to add another provider to the schedule. The length of employment varies with locum tenens and can be as short as a few days or as long as months at a time. If you find a facility is a good fit, you may be able continue working as a locum for that company or it may even turn into a permanent placement position.

There will be much more information on the different types of nurse practitioner job opportunities in chapter seven. However, I just wanted to mention some of the various options available to show you a little bit about the profession and hopefully get you excited about what the future entails. I've also included in the appendix an extensive list of NP employment resources to help with your job search.

Job Outlook

As stated earlier, it is estimated that there are over 234,000 NPs licensed in the United States (NP Fact Sheet, 2017), with more people choosing to become nurse practitioners every year. Fortunately for you as a future NP, there are no shortages of nurse practitioner jobs, and finding work won't necessarily be a problem. Not only is the job outlook incredible, but the U.S. News & World Report of the 100 Best Jobs of 2018 ranked NPs as #4! You can check out this list at https://money.usnews.com/careers/best-jobs/rankings/the-100-best-jobs.

Aside from the fact that there are thousands of jobs available, changing outdated state laws will also allow NPs to have more autonomy to manage their patients. As collaborative agreements fall to the wayside and restrictions are eliminated, NPs are now practicing more than ever to the full extent of their training. NPs will continue to be in high demand as they provide much-needed services and high-quality patient care.

Nurse practitioners are also at the forefront for providing care to the influx of newly insured patients who now have insurance due to the Affordable Care Act. This increase in patients coupled with the aging Baby Boomer population ensures that nurse practitioners will continue to be needed throughout the nation. There is a critical shortage of healthcare providers in this country, especially in the primary care sector, and nurse practitioners continue to be a part of the solution.

Nurse Practitioner Salaries

Apart from having a great job outlook, nurse practitioners also bring home a robust salary. In 2017, the mean salary for a full-time nurse practitioner was just over 105,000 (NP Fact Sheet, 2017). However, many of my NP colleagues make much more than this annually. As far as payment goes you may be paid salary or hourly and the amount you will receive depends on your specialty, experience, education, and where you work. You may also receive additional compensation for seeing more patients. In short, if you decide to work as a nurse practitioner you will most likely have opportunities for employment making an above-average salary for life.

As you have read in this chapter, nurse practitioners have a long, rich professional history and continue to make headway in the workforce today. If you are already a practicing NP, then these facts should come as no surprise. However, for those of you who are interested in the profession or are currently in a nurse practitioner program, this is a very exciting time to be part of one of the fastest-growing and most in-demand professions of our time.

I hope that this chapter has gotten you excited about your journey to becoming a nurse practitioner. There is definitely a lot to be enthusiastic about when pursuing this career, and the future holds endless possibilities. Now that you understand the history and role of an NP, let's move on to chapter two to find out how to become a nurse practitioner!

References

Bishop, C. S. (2012). Advanced practitioners are not mid-level providers. *Journal of the Advanced Practitioner in Oncology, 3*(5). doi: 10.6004/jadpro.2012.3.5.1

Buppert, C. (2008). *Nurse practitioner's business practice and legal guide*. Burlington, MA: Jones & Bartlett Learning.

Committee on the Robert Wood Johnson Foundation Initiative on the Future of Nursing, at the Institute of Medicine. (2011). *The future of nursing: Leading change, advancing health*. Washington, D. C.: National Academies Press.

Historical Timeline. aanp.org. Retrieved June 3, 2017 from https://www.aanp.org/all-about-nps/historical-timeline

NP Fact Sheet. aanp.org. Retrieved June 3, 2017 from https://www.aanp.org/all-about-nps/np-fact-sheet

O'Brien, J. M. (2003). How nurse practitioners obtained provider status: Lessons for pharmacists. *American Journal of Health System Pharmacy, 60*(22), 2301–2307.

Scope of Practice for Nurse Practitioners. (n.d.). American Assosciation of Nurse Practitioners. Retrieved November 18, 2017 from https://www.aanp.org/images/documents/publications/scopeofpractice.pdf

Stanik-Hutt, J., Newhouse, R. P., White, K. M., Johantgen, M., Bass, E. B., Zangaro, G., Weiner, J. P. (2013). The quality and effectiveness of care provided by nurse practitioners. *The Journal for Nurse Practitioners, 9*(8), 492–500. doi:10.1016/j.nurpra.2013.07.004.

Swan, M., Ferguson, S., Chang, A., Larson, E., & Smaldone, A. (2015). Quality of primary care by advanced practice nurses: A systematic review. *International Journal for Quality in Health Care, 27*(5), 396–404. doi:10.1093/intqhc/mzv054

· 2 ·

HOW TO GET ACCEPTED INTO A NURSE PRACTITIONER PROGRAM

To accomplish great things, you must not only act, but also dream, not only plan, but also believe.

—Anatole France

As you have learned in chapter one, the nurse practitioner profession is incredibly diverse and continues to evolve. Now that you have a better understanding about the history of the profession and the role of a nurse practitioner, it is now time to focus on how you will achieve your goal to actually become a nurse practitioner. There are many roads leading to a career as an NP, and each individual's life path is different. Hence, the way you achieve this goal will be different than others. How I became an NP will be much different than how you will become an NP. I encourage you not to compare yourself with other future NPs and focus on your end goal of becoming a nurse practitioner.

This chapter is dedicated to helping you get accepted into a nurse practitioner program. The following pages will guide you in creating a strong application that will assist you in getting accepted into the school of your dreams. The contents of this chapter will also help you choose between programs if you are offered multiple acceptance letters. Although multiple acceptances can be a testament to just how strong an applicant you are, they can also create confusion and self-doubt as to which program is best for you. This chapter will offer guidance on how to find the best fit for you and hopefully lead you to the school and program that you will enjoy.

Regardless of where you are on the road to becoming a nurse practitioner, this chapter will offer you practical guidance throughout the process. Even if you've already been accepted into a program, I encourage you to continue reading as there will still be relevant information that you may find helpful.

How to Get Accepted into a Nurse Practitioner Program

Whether you think you can or you think you can't, either way you are right.
—Henry Ford

I love the above quote because I truly believe in what Henry Ford is saying; regardless of whether you think you can or cannot achieve a certain goal you are correct, as your thoughts create your world. I could write an entire book about my experiences with the law of attraction, the power of visualization, and manifesting my dreams. From personal experience, I have seen these things happen in my own life. Regardless of what I say, you will need to come to these conclusions (either agreeing or disagreeing) on your own. Nonetheless, I'd like to share my experience with these concepts prior to even getting accepted into my nurse practitioner program.

While I was applying to various nurse practitioner programs I created my first ever vision board, which I looked at daily. For those of you not familiar with a vision board it's a poster board or box on which you paste images and phrases about what you want in your life. My vision board had images of New York City (as I mentioned before I wanted to attend Columbia University), words about nurses and nurse practitioners, and basically anything that I wanted out of the next phase of my life. While looking at my vision board I'd imagine what it was like to be a student at Columbia while living in Manhattan. After months of positive visualizations and dreaming of being an NP student, lo and behold yours truly was accepted into Columbia University School of Nursing. I do believe that aside from all of the hard work and dedication that it took to get into an NP program, staying positive and focusing on what I wanted (and not on what I didn't want) made all of the difference.

Since my first successful vision board, I've used vision boards and the power of positive thinking in various aspects of my life and have always been astounded by what it brings me. After my successful NYC vision board experience, I decided it was time for another vision board for the next phase of my life. After I had graduated my NP program and was applying to various positions, I made another vision board, this time of Hawaii. I had recently interviewed for a position in the Aloha State and was really hoping that I would get the job. I put images of Hawaii, sea turtles swimming in the Pacific, and palm trees on the beach all over the board and placed it in a location that I would see every day. And what do you know? I received the job in Hawaii where I spent the next two years living and working as an NP.

Go ahead and give the vision board a try; you have nothing to lose. If you need inspiration you can browse Google or Pinterest. If vision boards and affirmations aren't your cup of tea I still suggest remaining positive and believing in yourself during the application process. This can be a challenging time when you are balancing patience and perhaps anxiety while waiting to hear from admissions offices. Negativity will only hinder you and may even create self-fulfilling prophecies. So my advice to you is to stay positive.

This chapter may seem challenging as there is a lot of information within it, but I want you to try and remain as upbeat as you can. You've made it this far in your career, and deciding to become a nurse practitioner is no easy feat. Stay strong in your conviction that if becoming a nurse practitioner is something you really want, you will achieve it.

The Application Process

With an increasing number of individuals deciding to become nurse practitioners, competition to get into programs can be fierce. I remember all the emotions that I was feeling while applying to multiple universities. Anxiety, stress, self-doubt, and excitement followed me during the application process. Questions ran through my head such as, will I get in? What if I don't get in? Will I succeed? And once I am accepted, how will I pay for it all? Did I choose the right school? You may be having similar thoughts and feelings during the application process, or you may be one of those relaxed people (like my husband, for example) who goes with the flow of life and is confident that the right thing will happen at the right time. I'm getting there, but this definitely wasn't my mindset during the application process! Regardless of how you are feeling, applying to a nurse practitioner program (especially if you apply to multiple schools) can be an arduous process, both physically and mentally.

I'd like to begin by saying that admissions requirements vary by each school and program. The information presented in this chapter is a generalization of what you may come across during the application process. However, you need to do your due diligence and check with each individual school/program for specific admissions requirements. For example, some NP programs may require additional courses while others may require an interview. It all depends on the school's individual requirements, which should be posted on their admissions website. Although each program's specific admissions requirements may vary slightly, admissions committees are basically looking for similar criteria when reviewing your application.

To get more understanding on what exactly admissions are looking for, I questioned one admissions advisor about the most important part of the application. She informed me that they generally don't look at applications in pieces but in their entirety. As the applicant is generally viewed more holistically, if there is some area where you are weaker, such as your grade point average (GPA), you may be able to boost that with a stronger component from another section. Now granted that was one admissions advisor from one university; however, I think she makes a valid point that by having a strong, well-rounded application you will be an overall stronger applicant.

To simplify things as best as I could I've broken down the application process into individual sections so you can see what may be required of you prior to submitting yours. Again, it is highly advised to review each program's requirements prior to applying to make sure you have met all necessary requirements. You may even want to start a spreadsheet on what each school requires as this may help keep you organized and potentially save you a lot of time in the future.

Prerequisite Courses

There are generally several prerequisite courses that must be completed prior to starting your nurse practitioner program. Depending on how many science courses you took as an undergraduate, you may need to take additional prerequisite courses as part of admissions requirements. This is one of the admissions requirements that I suggest you take a look at first as it may take you a year or two (depending on your schedule) to complete all the required prerequisite courses prior to even applying to your program.

When I first decided I wanted to be a nurse practitioner I wasn't sure what school I wanted to attend much less where I would even be applying. However, I did my research early on and found the courses that many schools were requiring prior to entry. Since I didn't know where I would be applying, I took additional courses that I didn't need. Looking back, although I may not have needed to take as many courses as I did, it provided me with more options of potential schools to apply to.

Many schools will still allow you to apply to their program while finishing these courses, but admission is dependent on successfully completing them and submitting final transcripts once the course has been completed. Classes you may need prior to entering your NP program (in addition to your undergraduate courses) may include but are not limited to: anatomy and physiology I and II, microbiology, statistics, nutrition, and chemistry. It is also important to keep in mind that many science courses are required to be current. If you took these courses many years ago you may have to repeat them if they are too old. You can verify if you need to repeat these courses with your program's office of admissions. Again, make sure to look at your program's specific requirements to ensure you complete all required courses.

Grade Point Average (GPA)

Your grade point average (GPA) is the average grade you have received over a given period of time. GPA can definitely factor into a decision on whether to admit you to an NP program, and many students often worry about their GPA negatively affecting their application. Although you may have graduated with your undergraduate degree years ago, that D you received in your undergraduate English class may still be haunting you. However, admissions committees do realize that people change over time and become more mature and far better students than they were earlier in their career.

Your GPA does not include just your grades from your undergraduate degree but your prerequisite courses as well. This is great news to someone who had less than average grades as an undergraduate, as they can now show that they are focused and dedicated by doing well during their prerequisite courses. This definitely works in your favor, so don't get too discouraged if your undergraduate grades weren't fantastic as you now have the chance to do well on your prerequisite courses. Your GPA for your prerequisites can sometimes overshadow your undergraduate GPA as they are the basic core science courses you are required to take prior to being admitted into an NP program. By doing well in your prerequisite courses, regardless of your undergraduate GPA, you are definitely giving the GPA portion of your application even more strength.

Your GPA is submitted to each school you are applying to in the form of a transcript, usually an official transcript. This may be required to be sent directly from your previous academic institution(s) or in an official letter that is sealed and sent with the rest of your application. If the latter is how you will be submitting your transcript, do not open it as this may render your official transcript invalid! If you are still in the process of taking prerequisite courses after submitting your application, you will need to send in your transcript as soon as your grades are posted, for verification of course completion.

My undergraduate GPA was okay but definitely not anything to be exceptionally proud of. I took almost two years of prerequisite science courses as part of the admissions requirements for my NP program. This allowed me to bring up my grades and prove to schools that I was serious about my education. If I can do it so can you; it just requires patience and dedication to complete all necessary courses.

If science isn't your strong suit don't get discouraged. I thought it wasn't mine either. Despite my mother being a science teacher, I was never really interested in science prior to my NP journey. Now I am fascinated with the mechanics of the human body and really enjoy medicine. At the beginning these courses may be challenging; however, with time you will become more familiar with the topics and may even enjoy them! Use your resources, form study groups with your classmates, get tutoring, and of course spend ample amounts of time studying on your own. Basically, find the best study methods that will help you to succeed.

Personal Statement

The personal statement requirement of your application is a way for you to differentiate yourself from other applicants and to use your own words to bring life to your application. Although schools vary in what they want you to write about, essentially you will be explaining the reason you chose to become a nurse practitioner, and perhaps why you want to attend that specific school. From what I've been told, a well-written personal statement is one of the strongest pieces that you can add to your NP program application. The personal statement gives your application personality and your voice, passions, and goals can really shine through. This is one of the ways that you are able to distinguish yourself from your co-applicants.

Make sure you read carefully what your program is asking from you in your statement. Do not write about something completely different than the topic required for the personal statement. You will do yourself no favors by writing on something completely off topic, regardless of how well written the statement is. I suggest putting a lot of time and thought into this piece as it may mean the difference between acceptance and rejection. Here are a few suggestions that may help guide you on what to write about in your personal statement.

- Why do you want to be a nurse practitioner?
- Was there any particular experience that led you on the path to become a nurse practitioner?
- If you are currently an RN, why are you interested in becoming an NP?
- Why do you want to attend that specific school? If you would like to write more on this topic I highly suggest researching the school and pulling out key reasons that attracted you to that specific program. Reasons to attend a specific program run the gamut from clinical experience, location, faculty, and overall reputation of the program.
- Previous health-related experiences.
- Previous personal experiences.
- Family member experience with a health-related issue.
- Issues you have seen with the healthcare system and why you would like to be an agent for change.
- If you had a former profession prior to deciding to become an NP, what made you decide to leave your old job and pursue a health-related career?
- What kind of patient population interests you?

Writing a solid personal statement will not only help strengthen your application, but it may also be beneficial when applying for scholarships as many scholarships also require personal statements and/or essays. You can use one essay and tweak it for different application purposes. This will save you a lot of time and energy in the future.

Recently I've seen that some schools require a video essay in addition to a written personal statement. If this is the case, make sure you practice what you're going to say, dress professionally, and take more than one video to ensure the highest quality will be sent to the school. Again, make sure to discuss on the video what is requested of you. Have fun with it. It's a great way to make yourself shine!

Essay

Some programs will require an essay in addition to a personal statement. You may even be required to write more than one essay as part of your application. Essays differ from personal statements as the personal statement is about you, while an essay can be about a variety of topics. You may be given a statement to respond to or be asked to write on a certain subject. Or you may be given a question that you have to answer. Although essays tend to be less personal than the statement, you can still use your voice to bring life and add personality to your essay.

> *Tip*. If writing is not one of your strong suits I suggest getting assistance from a friend, family, or colleague to review your work and edit it for you once you have written it. My cousin is a great writer and helped edit many of my statements, papers, and scholarship essays after I had written them. This helped me immensely and I'm very grateful that she helped with this.

Graduate Record Exam (GRE)

The graduate record exam, more commonly known as the GRE, is an exam for students who wish to pursue graduate coursework within a certain field. This exam tests your verbal, quantitative, and analytic reasoning. This will most likely be a requirement for your entrance into your nurse practitioner program. To find out more about the exam and register for a test, visit www.ets.org/gre/revised_general/about.

When applying to NP school many of my colleagues were incredibly nervous about taking the GRE. I don't remember the exam in great detail nor do I remember my score, but don't get too freaked out about taking it. During your time in your NP program you will have to take many tests. Just think of this as the first of many you will eventually have to complete.

I suggest that you give yourself ample time to study for the GRE so you don't have to take it again. There are many great study resources to help you prepare for the examination, and I highly advise using some sort of study tool to best prepare you for the exam. This is a test you don't want to take twice, so make studying a priority!

Letters of Recommendation

As part of the application process you will typically be asked to supply two or three letters of recommendation from people who know you professionally such as former supervisors, professors, or peers. Family members and friends are generally not permitted to write these letters for you. These references are essentially vouching for you based on your previous work and interactions with them. Make sure to choose people who have only positive things to say about you. This may seem like a no-brainer; however, I've heard of plenty of stories about people getting bad-mouthed on a letter of recommendation. Why they would ask someone who would write them a less than spectacular recommendation beats me, so my advice is to choose wisely!

Depending on where you apply, each letter of recommendation may be a completely different format. Letters of recommendation templates run the gamut and there should be specific instructions on how they will be submitted to the school. Some letters are to be filled out in a pre-existing paper question-naire format, while others must be filled out electronically. Some schools will ask for a letter on official letterhead that does not require the person to answer any specific questions, but rather to write freely about their experiences with you.

With all of these options available to submit just one component of your application, I recommend you stay highly organized and keep track of which letter goes to what school. If you are applying to multiple schools and feel that the people you have asked to write your letter of recommendation may be overwhelmed by filling out ten different forms, consider having one or two individuals for backup who can assist you with this process. If the letter comes directly to you to include in your application, I suggest scanning it (if it's in a non-sealed envelope) to save, as you never know when you'll need to use it again.

Most importantly, always remember to thank the people who wrote you a letter of recommendation. They are providing a much-needed service to you and could be the reason why you are accepted into a specific program. I usually will send a handwritten card or thank you email after they have submitted the letters. A little thank you can go a long way, and you never know when you may need another letter of recommendation in the future.

Tip. Be sure to give the people you ask to provide letters of recommendation plenty of time to fill out the appropriate paperwork. I recommend having this be one of the first things that you address when you start applying to nurse practitioner programs. This ensures that you give the writer plenty of time to reflect on all of your good qualities without feeling pressured with a deadline. I also recommend giving them a deadline way in advance of the actual deadline, just in case they lag in completing it.

If you are having problems receiving the letter after a predetermined date, politely send a reminder email letting them know the deadline is arriving and that if they are unable to submit it in time to kindly let you know and you will ask someone else. Most people are more than happy to do this for you, but often it gets pushed to the bottom of the pile. It's your job to remind them (nicely and patiently) to get it done!

Resume/Curriculum Vitae (CV)

Your resume or CV often must be submitted with your completed application. This is another way to highlight all the different experiences you have had that you were unable to relay in other sections of your application. Include all relevant information and make sure to put extra emphasis on certain areas that may differentiate you from other candidates. This may include awards and recognitions, clinical experience, volunteer experience, or anything else that you have accomplished. Even if what you have done has nothing to do with nursing and medicine, if it's something you are proud of accomplishing, put it in there. Nurse practitioner programs like diversity, so just because you think that the award you won for planting trees isn't important, it doesn't mean the admissions committee will agree with you.

Tip. I recommend printing out your resume and proofreading it as a hardcopy (do this also with your personal statement, essays, and any other written document you will be submitting). Many times, errors are overlooked as we are so used to reading text on the computer screen. To have something physically in your hand increases the likelihood you will pick up on something previously missed. After you read it to yourself and have made the appropriate corrections, read it out loud as well to recheck for anything you may have missed. I also suggest having another person read it, ensuring all possible mistakes are corrected. I once made the unfortunate mistake of writing on my resume that I wanted to work with "*undeserved* communities" instead of "underserved communities." A recruiter for a company I was interviewing with noticed the mistake and kindly brought it to my attention. I still cringe at how many of my misspelled resumes were circulating through cyberspace.

Work/Life Experience

This section can also be included under the resume/CV and/ or personal statement portion of your application if the program you are applying to does not include a separate section for this piece. However, I've decided to talk about work/life experience as its own entity because I think it is also a very strong part of your application that enables you to highlight your own individual strengths, experiences, and uniqueness.

If you are applying to your NP program with previous nursing experience, this is a great place to highlight all the clinical settings where you've worked. If there is a specific patient that sticks out in your mind, provide details about how you took care of that individual or what made the experience so special. Maybe you saw something while working as an RN that inspired you to pursue a career as an NP. Perhaps there was an injustice you witnessed that made you want to be in a better place to advocate for your patients. Regardless of what you choose to write about, I suggest speaking from your heart because the readers of your application will know if you're being authentic or not.

On the other hand if you are new to the profession and don't have any previous clinical nursing experience, do not fret as you can still list previous experiences that are relevant. I liken this to the transferrable skills that people often talk about when applying for a job; when you don't have the specific skill set but have other skills that are relevant to the position they can be transferrable into your new role. For example, volunteer experience is a great way to highlight your life experiences. Even though you may not have been working with patients, you still dealt with other people and worked toward the greater good of something. In my case, since I was applying to the direct entry bachelor of science in nursing program and didn't have any previous RN experience, I focused on my work as a health volunteer in Cameroon during my time as a Peace Corps Volunteer. This allowed me to talk about the work I did in the health setting, even though my clinical experience at that point was basically zero.

The beauty of having a diverse applicant pool is that while you are attending your nurse practitioner program you will meet so many people with incredibly diverse backgrounds and experiences. Most of my NP friends were not nurses prior to applying to their NP program; they came from all sorts of backgrounds including corporate America. Learning and networking with your fellow classmates will only make you a stronger and a better nurse practitioner. Don't assume that just because you don't have previous experience working in a hospital or clinic that you are a weaker applicant. Focus on your strengths and transferable skills from previous experiences that you've had, and turn these experiences into an advantage.

Interview

Certain nurse practitioner programs require interviews while others do not. Interviews can be in person, on the phone, or via video chat. Only one of the schools that I applied to required an interview, and this was done by phone. I thought the interview went well, despite being incredibly nervous, and I was offered admission into the program, but decided not to attend. An interview can be a great way for you to show just how interested you are in a specific school, and you can explain exactly why you want to be an NP. Many times, applicants can shine during a conversation in a way they just can't on paper. If you have an interview as part of your admissions requirements make sure to give yourself plenty of time to prepare, similar to a job interview. I suggest having a friend or family member practice interviewing you to best prepare. Also, if you have a Skype or a face-to-face interview make sure to dress professionally!

International Students

If you are an international applicant who graduated from a university in which courses were not taught in English, you may need to sit for the TOEFL exam. Short for Test of English as a Foreign Language, TOEFL is a test for non native speakers of English to demonstrate their English proficiency for academic purposes, specifically at the university level. For more information on the exam you can visit www.ets.org/toefl.

Furthermore, if you are an international student you will have to submit transcripts that differ from the standard U.S. transcript. You may be required to have your transcripts evaluated by an agency that is accredited by the National Association of Credential Evaluation Services, or NACES for short. Remember, specific requirements vary by school and if you are an international applicant I encourage you to contact the school's admissions office if you have any questions about what is required of you. There may be an office at your school specifically dedicated to international students, which can be a great resource for you. Some schools even give priority on-campus housing to international students!

As an international student, you are not eligible for federal student loans. However, there are a variety of other resources you can take advantage of to fund your education. These include private lenders, scholarships, and grants. There will be much more detail on financial aid resources in chapter four. I also encourage you to check with your school's financial aid office to see if they have any additional funding resources for international students.

Application Fees and Deadlines

The programs to which you apply will most likely charge you an application fee as part of the application requirements. Application fees can range in price, so make sure to factor this into your application as costs can add up. Additionally, do not forget that application deadlines for each school vary so it's important to make sure your completed application has arrived by this deadline. You don't want to forfeit your chance as a potential student just because your application was late, so please plan accordingly!

Reviewing Your Application

Once you have gathered everything you need to apply to the nurse practitioner programs that you wish to attend, you will need to do a complete review of your application in its entirety. Look diligently for any areas of weakness in your application and then do your best to try and bolster them. I suggest really taking time to make a solid, strong application; you don't want to have to go through the entire application process only to be rejected due to a preventable error. Applying to NP school is time consuming and can be quite pricey. Similar to taking the GRE, you want the application process to be a one-time experience only!

If there is an informational session or open house that is being held for an NP program you are interested in, I suggest attending. This will give you a chance to ask questions about your application and about the program in general. This also gives you the chance to meet with faculty and get a feel for the campus and what being a student there may be like. Remember, just because you may not think you have a strong application does not mean that the admissions committee will agree with you. Keep your spirits high and realize that many other applicants may have less than perfect applications as well.

If you think that one or more parts of your application may bar you from admittance, there are ways to strengthen them. To determine how strong your application is, use Table 2.1 to evaluate which components of your application are strengths and which are weaknesses that may require more effort from you. Then revisit your application and make any needed changes that will further strengthen your application. For example, if you feel that your resume is weak and needs a little boost, perhaps getting it looked at professionally will help make it a stronger component for your application.

As you have read throughout this chapter it is obvious that preparing for and applying to nurse practitioner programs is no small task. During this time, you may be juggling work, taking prerequisite courses, studying for the GRE, researching schools, and putting together a solid application all at the same time! You may also be vigorously applying for various scholarships and looking into different financial aid packages. The application process may require months if not years of your time to complete all required components. Before getting too overwhelmed, take a deep breath and realize that the application process may be similar to your time as a nurse practitioner student when you will be balancing a seemingly mountainous array of tasks at the same time. You could look at the application process as a training course for what is to come once you've begun your program!

As I've stated above, this is a process you only want to go through once, so I suggest preparing your applications in advance of when they are due. Give yourself enough time to research schools, gather all necessary components of your application, and apply to each institution. I strongly suggest that you do not wait for the month before your applications are due to start the application process. Time management is not only essential to applying to NP programs, but it is also a necessity to successfully completing your NP program. You'll thank yourself when you're not up until midnight the night before an application is due scrambling to finish!

Now that you have a better understanding of what is required of you as an applicant for NP school, let's now switch gears to chapter three. In this next chapter, you will learn about the different ways to enter into your NP program, how to decide which programs you will be applying to, and where you will eventually decide to attend.

Table 2.1. Nurse Practitioner Application Review.

Application component	Strength (+ or -)	What can be done to make this piece stronger?
Prerequisite Courses		
GPA		
Personal Statement		
GRE Score		
Letters of Recommendation		
Work/Life Experience		
Resume/CV		
Essay		
Interview		
Other		

Source: Author.

· 3 ·

DECIDING ON A NURSE PRACTITIONER PROGRAM

It is in your moments of decision that your destiny is shaped.

—Tony Robbins

I am a big fan of Tony Robbins and his messages. Through his work and his books, he is able to better the lives of many people. I also love the above quote because it's completely true. Your life is all about a series of decisions you will make, both large and small, that will shape your future. While I was applying to NP programs I too had to make a quick decision, which I believe altered the course of my life.

I had applied to Columbia's early acceptance program but hadn't gotten in, and I was fearful that I wouldn't be admitted during the regular admissions period. During this time, I was also offered acceptance into another NP program in upstate New York. Upon being accepted to this other program, I had a limited amount of time to pay the $500 non-refundable deposit to secure my seat. As I still hadn't heard from Columbia, I decided to mail in the money for the other program after holding out until the very last day. My plan was to drop off the check at the post office before heading to work.

Why I had to go all the way to the post office to mail the check is also puzzling as I could have mailed it from my apartment complex; however, looking back on it I assume this too was part of the divine plan. That day as I drove to the post office my intuition suddenly told me not to mail in the check and so I headed to work instead. I knew that by doing this I was most likely forfeiting my chance of acceptance, but something just didn't feel right. However, as Lady Fate always intervenes at the correct time, when I got to work I checked my email and guess what? I was accepted into Columbia! Had I not listened to my gut I would have lost that $500 and perhaps questioned attending Columbia as I had already paid money toward another program. It was that quick decision I made to not send in the money that helped me in the end and saved me $500!

Different Ways to Enter into a Nurse Practitioner Program

This chapter is dedicated to helping you decide which nurse practitioner programs you will be applying to, as well as provide assistance in selecting the best fit program for you. Researching and writing this chapter was much more complicated than I thought it would be. While exploring different nurse practitioner programs, I came to realize just how many available options there were to someone interested in becoming a nurse practitioner. Therefore, I've decided to break it down piece by piece and make this topic as straightforward as possible.

Although there are hundreds of nurse practitioner programs available to you, they vary from each other in distinct ways. Programs have various admissions requirements and not all programs will offer the same degree once you graduate. For example, some programs require a BSN prior to entering, while others award you a BSN upon completion. Certain programs offer an accelerated BSN program while others do not, and you may even receive a post-master's certificate once you complete your program. With so many options available it can be quite confusing!

While previously you were able to become a nurse practitioner with a master's degree without needing to receive your doctorate degree, due to consensus, the American Association of Nurse Practitioners (AANP) has decided to eliminate the master's degree and go straight to the doctorate level degree—the Doctor of Nursing Practice (DNP) degree. Although this hasn't taken place in every NP program just yet, numerous programs have already adopted this change and will continue to transition out the master's in favor of the DNP degree.

Although it may seem challenging to try and understand all of the different programs, there are basically two ways to enter into an NP program. Essentially, you will enter into your program with a bachelor's degree in an unrelated field or you will enter your program as a registered nurse having already completed your Bachelor of Science in Nursing (BSN).

Nurse Practitioner from a Non-Nursing Background

If you do not already hold a BSN you will most likely be applying to a direct entry program. The direct entry admissions programs are designed for students who already have a bachelor's degree in another subject and who have decided to pursue a career in nursing. This is typically referred to as a "second career"; however, I've met several students who started their direct entry program right after their undergraduate degree, thus nursing was their first career.

There are both direct entry BSN and MSN programs available. There are certain programs in which you will receive both a bachelor's and master's degree. There are also other programs where you will receive just a master's degree. As stated above, some schools will require you to have a doctorate in order to become a nurse practitioner; thus you may not get your master's degree at all, but your DNP instead. As there are so many different programs and schools available and each is different, I cannot get too specific and have to generalize. Nevertheless, the outcome is the same as you will complete your program as a nurse practitioner with one or more degrees (I finished mine with three degrees). If the direct entry program is what you are looking for then you are in luck as many schools offer this option.

Nurse Practitioner from BSN Degree

If you are already a registered nurse and hold a BSN, entering into an NP program is much more straightforward. You will most likely still need to complete prerequisite courses prior to entering your program, and the application process is similar to those who do not yet having a nursing degree. You will definitely have to hold an active RN license in the state where you are applying. Upon graduation, you will receive a master's or doctorate degree or both.

Accelerated Nurse Practitioner Programs

You may also come across the term "accelerated" while researching potential nurse practitioner programs. Accelerated programs are exactly this; they are quick-paced programs that allow you to obtain a BSN or MSN degree. This is done at a much faster speed than an average program. These programs can be incredibly rigorous, and if you decide to attend an accelerated program, be prepared to study. During this time, you will be immersed in nursing theory, pharmacology, clinical rotations, and everything in between. If you are an in an accelerated BSN program you may also be taking master's level classes concomitantly with your BSN courses.

As I was a student of a direct entry accelerated BSN program I can personally attest to the rigor of the curriculum. While some of my friends were going out every weekend, I was spending a lot of my time at the library. Since I was new to the whole healthcare profession, everything I learned was a novelty to me, and I was incredibly inexperienced. I remember my first day of clinical as a nursing student in a prominent New York City hospital. There I was in my navy blue scrubs and shiny white nursing shoes (I still cringe that I had to wear them) with exactly zero clinical experience. I went into my first patient room to take vitals…simple enough, right? Not so much. I proceeded to put the blood pressure cuff on the patient unknowingly inside out, and as it began to inflate it popped right off the patient's arm. The patient looked at me point blank and asked, "Do you know what you're doing?" Um, no, I did not and I couldn't even fake that I had any idea that I did. I sheepishly exited the patient's room hoping to not have another major fail for the rest of the day.

Different Types of Nurse Practitioner Programs

Now that we have discussed the different ways to enter into an NP program, let's switch gears to review the different types of NP programs available. Nurse practitioner programs come in a variety of forms with many different options available for incoming students. There is a plethora of specialties, subspecialties, and certificate programs available to choose from. There are part-time programs and there are full-time programs. There are programs held primarily online and those held primarily on campus. There are also programs that combine both an online and an on-campus curriculum, often referred to as hybrid programs. There are accelerated programs, direct entry programs, bachelor's, master's and doctoral programs, which I have previously mentioned. You get it,—there are a lot of program options to choose from!

As you begin your search into where you want to apply, try not to become too overwhelmed with all the different programs and options. There may even be some confusion surrounding some of the terms used to describe your potential program. As you start to narrow your search you'll find some programs won't interest or pertain to you, while others will capture your attention. Hopefully the contents of this chapter will make that process easier. Now let's get started on the various nurse practitioner programs available to you.

On Campus

Since there are so many options available I thought it best to begin your search by deciding how you want to attend class—either on campus or online. I can't personally speak to taking a program that is completely online, as the majority of my education took place on campus with limited online content. However, I can personally attest to the benefits of being in an on-campus program. For me, this type of program fit my learning style much better than an online program would have. Being in person allowed me to connect face to face with my professors, and I was able to get to know my classmates really well. I felt that my learning was enhanced as I was constantly surrounded by fellow students discussing recently learned content, studying, or reviewing difficult material with my professors. As I didn't have a relatively strong science background prior to starting my NP studies, I learned an incredible amount just by spending time with my peers.

I also really enjoyed getting to know the other students. From late night study sessions to celebrating the end of a semester, my classmates were with me every step of the way. Many of these people have become some of my closest friends and I still speak with them on a regular basis. Personally, it would have been a lot harder to make it through my program without my classmates and friends by my side. They were also the only group of people who personally understood what I was going through during my program. Yes, I could complain to my family about the rigorousness of what I was studying, but they never understood exactly what I meant. My classmates on the other hand were in the trenches with me and could personally attest to the ups and downs that I was feeling as they were also experiencing them.

Attending an on-campus program also means you will most likely will be surrounded by campus activities. My school put on a lot of activities for its students and there was always something going on. In my free time I'd teach yoga (I'm also a registered yoga teacher) or take yoga classes that were exclusive to students. I'd meet my friends at student events where we could unwind and not think about classwork. I also participated in volunteer events through my school, which was a great way to practice my newly learned clinical skills and get to know the community. These activities brought in a lightness to the student experience and I'm grateful to have participated in them. Your school may offer similar opportunities for its students and you also may be able to participate in activities comparable to those that I partook in.

For me, being in an on-campus program was also incredibly convenient as I lived blocks away from the school and library. If I needed to print, scan, or get documents it took me only a few minutes to get to where I needed to go. I could meet with my professors and get to study groups without much notice, and could go home and crash right after a long day without a long commute home. I do admit that this convenience was mostly due to location since I was so close to school without actually living on campus. On the other hand, I had a lot of friends who commuted to campus for class and this was not convenient for them at all. Some would spend two to three hours a day commuting! I highly suggest that if you decide to attend an on-campus program you live near the school that you will be attending. You will save yourself a lot of time and stress by doing so.

Another great aspect of participating in an on-campus program was that it was a great way to network and create professional connections. From job fairs to residency informational sessions, being on campus allowed me to participate in these events and get to know others in the field aside from people whom I had met at Columbia.

As you can see, an on-campus program has a lot of perks; however, you will ultimately decide which program works best for your life. I really enjoyed the on-campus student experience and although once I graduated there was great joy in all that I had accomplished, there was also sadness at saying good-bye to those I'd come to know and love so well.

Online

On the other side of the spectrum are online programs, which have become an increasingly popular option for NP students. I have met many students who prefer online learning over attending classes in person, as it fits their learning style better and they can learn at their own pace. Some students choose online programs so they don't have to move to attend a program and thus uproot their life. Others may have a full-time job that only permits them to go to class after work hours, thus they are able to both keep their job and also minimize their debt. Attending classes online definitely has the convenience factor as a benefit and is something to consider when deciding on which program you will choose.

While I was writing this section of my book I spoke with a friend of mine who has been an RN for years and who was just accepted into an FNP online program in the south. She is a full-time mom of three young children under the age of five, works a part-time job, and was now beginning a new chapter in her life and career. She had just finished her on-campus orientation and was very excited about how supportive both the staff and fellow students were. Despite it being an online program, she felt she would be very connected to her classmates and faculty throughout the program. She told me that during orientation she got a few phone numbers from her classmates, and they started a group study guide together. She was also invited to join a class Facebook group, thus creating more camaraderie with her peers. She was really excited about the upcoming program. A few months later right before her first semester finals, I checked in with my friend again to see how her program was going, and to find out if she still felt supported by the staff and classmates. She stated that she still felt connected despite being in a virtual classroom, and despite the rigorousness of the program was able to keep up with the pace.

Even though a program may be online it can't be 100% online because there are clinical hours that you must complete in person. As part of your program requirements you will be working with a preceptor (someone you will shadow) in the clinical setting. Additionally, there are online programs that do require an in-person component at that school, which usually involves some sort of in-person testing. One of my nurse coworkers attended an online NP program on the East Coast but lived in Hawaii. He had to fly back East several times as a mandatory component of his program, though he was able to receive his clinical hours in his home state. Talk about a commute! Thank goodness for him this only involved a few trips and he wasn't required to have more face to face time. I highly suggest that prior to accepting an offer to an online NP program you make sure to find out exactly how much time is required of you in person.

Regardless of your circumstances, it is important to decide if attending an online program is the right learning style for you. If you've never taken online courses before, I encourage you to research techniques on how to be successful in an online program. It would be unfortunate if after you have begun your studies, you realized that you are unable to learn in this style. If attending an online nurse practitioner program interests you I encourage you to research schools with an online curriculum. Here is the link to the U.S. News & World Report rankings for best online graduate nursing schools: www.usnews.com/education/online-education/nursing/rankings.

Subspecialty Nurse Practitioner Programs

While you are applying to nurse practitioner programs, you may come across the option to choose a subspecialty to study in addition to the primary NP specialty that you have selected. A subspecialty program gives you the chance to learn about another aspect of healthcare in more depth than you would during your general NP studies. Typically, you will need to take additional courses in the area in which you will subspecialize, though you won't receive an additional degree. However, for certain subspecialties such as dermatology, there is no additional educational requirement, though you will need to complete a minimum number of hours working in dermatology prior to sitting for the board exam. There are several subspecialties under which you can become board certified.

Some of the subspecialty areas include but are not limited to HIV/AIDS, pediatric oncology, adult oncology, dermatology, and palliative care. You don't necessarily need to decide to subspecialize when you are applying to your program, as you may be able to choose this option while enrolled in your primary specialty curriculum. Subspecialty programs vary by school and may or may not be offered at your academic institution. Make sure to do your research into which school offers the subspecialty that you're interested in if you do in fact decide that you would like to subspecialize.

Post-Master's Certificate Programs

If you already hold your master's in nursing (MSN) you also have the option to obtain a post-master's certificate. These programs are designed for advanced practice registered nurses who wish to expand upon their knowledge or switch to another field in nursing. The post-master's certificate programs are not just for nurse practitioners, but for APRNs in general. For example, if you are already a family nurse practitioner and would like to broaden your pediatric knowledge, you can apply to a post-master's certificate program to also become a pediatric nurse practitioner. Or if you have your master's in nursing and are a practicing nurse-midwife, you can return to school to get your post-master's certificate in an NP specialty of your choice. Once you have received your post-master's certificate, then you will be able to sit for the board certification exam for that specialty. Many programs offer post-master's certificate programs, and I suggest considering this option if you already hold your MSN.

How to Determine Which Nurse Practitioner Schools You Should Apply to

Now that you are more familiar with the many types of nurse practitioner programs available, it is time to decide which schools you will actually be applying to. There are many quality schools to consider when deciding where you would like to complete your studies. It is important to really do your research into the school you may be attending and the location where you will be living for the next several years. If you are planning to move out of state for your program there is also a good chance you may land your first job in the state where you went to school. Thus, you will want to be extra selective when choosing the best fit school for you as you may end up there for a while.

Below is a list of frequently asked questions that will help guide you when you are trying to decide which school best fits your needs and where you will consider applying. You may also find the answers to some of these questions on the school's website. If you still have questions about the school and program, I suggest speaking to someone in the admissions department or a current student who can give you a student's perspective on what the program is like.

Nurse Practitioner Program Frequently Asked Questions

Do I prefer to live in a rural or urban setting?

This question is important because as they say, it's all about location, location, location! If you're from a small town, moving to a big city to complete your studies may seem overwhelming and perhaps something that you don't necessarily want to do. On the other hand, if you are a city person, moving to a rural and smaller community may not appeal to you either. Or maybe you want to stay where you are and don't want to move at all!

Prior to starting nursing school, I was overwhelmed at the thought of living in Manhattan. At the time, I was living in Arizona and the move from the calm and serenity of the desert to busy and bustling New York City was a huge deal for me. It's an understatement to say that I was very nervous. I was petrified! I didn't have much confidence that I would fit in, and I felt that I would be a small fish in a big pond. However, I completely proved myself wrong and ending up thriving in New York. It is important to consider where you want to live, but don't let self-limiting beliefs make the decision for you. If I had let my fear overcome me, I may not have had such an amazing experience.

Where will I get the best training?

As I did my training in New York City I thought that an urban environment was a great way to experience a plethora of different clinical rotations, clinics, and patient populations. Some of my rotations were in primary care, and some were very specialized such as an adult congenital heart rotation, which was incredibly fascinating. Since I attended a major academic institution associated with a hospital, I had the opportunity to see some pretty incredible things and felt that the big city was a great teacher.

However, after I graduated I moved to a rural setting and I learned a whole new skill set pertaining to a rural patient population in an underserved community. While working with this new patient population my knowledge increased exponentially and I learned new things daily. This included getting creative while managing my patients as they did not have easy access to specialists and/or other medical services that an urban patient population did. From working in one extreme to the other, I can honestly say that you will learn wherever you go, which is the very cool thing about this profession.

What percentage of students pass the NCLEX their first time?

The NCLEX, short for National Council Licensure Exam is the exam you must pass after completing your nursing studies in order to legally work as a registered nurse. This is applicable only if you are not yet a registered nurse prior to entering your program. If you enter into your NP program without being a registered nurse, you will have to take this exam prior to moving on with your studies.

You can often view a school's NCLEX pass rate posted online. The higher the percentage rate posted for a particular school means that students are being adequately prepared for the exam. The NCLEX is another exam that you only want to take one time, so I suggest you study and adequately prepare for it.

What schools have the specialty that I am considering pursuing?

If the school doesn't have the specialty you want to study, I suggest not applying there!

What schools have the subspecialty that I would like to study?

If you're interested in this option, be sure to check out the subspecialty programs that may be offered in addition to your curriculum. However, I wouldn't necessarily choose a program based on a subspecialty, as your scope of practice will be determined by your primary specialty.

Will I have to find my own preceptor or does the school provide preceptor placements?

I think this is a very important question to ask as it will determine how much work, if any, you will have to put in to finding a preceptor. A preceptor is someone who will mentor you during your clinical rotations and is usually another NP or physician. My program placed its students with preceptors, which was very helpful. However, we also had the option to choose our own preceptor if we met someone who was willing to take on this role. If your school requires you to find your own preceptor, you may want to ask them how this process works and if it's difficult to find a preceptor in your specialty. The school may have ways to assist students in this process, but I definitely think this question is worth inquiring about.

What kinds of financial aid does the school offer?

The answer to this question is very important to know because it may make or break your decision to attend a particular NP program. Many schools offer in-house scholarships to their students once they have been accepted into the program. There may also be additional scholarship money from the school's alumni organization. You may also be able to receive financial aid by working as a teaching assistant or by working on campus. It is important that you get information on how many awards are available and if you qualify for them. There will be more information on the various forms of financial aid later on in the text.

How much debt will I have once I complete the program?

It's good to get a ballpark figure as to how much you will owe after you complete your program. You may be able to get this information from the school's financial aid office.

What percentage of students who graduate pass the board certification exam on the first try?

Many schools post the pass rates online. It is a way to show how prepared their students are when they take their board examination.

What percentage of students who graduate have a job within six months? A year?

The goal of becoming a nurse practitioner is to get a nurse practitioner job once you graduate. The higher the number of students employed within a certain timeframe, the more likely that you will find a job within a similar period of time. For example, if 85% of students who graduate a program have a job within six months of graduation, this means you will most likely be hired within this period as well.

Am I able to work during the program?

I know that this was an important question for many students while I was a student, as working was a way to supplement student loans, helped cover living expenses, and provided a means to gain experience while working as a registered nurse. If you would like to work during your program, this may mean the difference between applying to one school or choosing another program that allows greater flexibility. I wasn't able to work during the direct entry BSN portion of my program due to the extremely rigorous curriculum. However, I did work through most of my master's and doctorate programs. I thought that working as an RN while concomitantly taking NP courses was very helpful as I was able to apply what I'd learned as a student directly to the clinical setting.

What kinds of extracurricular activities do students participate in?

Although your main priority is to be a student, you still need to have a life! My school had a lot of different activities and groups available to students, which were really fun to participate in. Extracurricular activities run the gamut and may mean anything from Friday afternoon craft events to holiday festivities to end of semester parties. For me, these social events took some of the stress out of daily life and I was able to relax with my peers without thinking about the next exam. If you would like to be involved in extracurricular activities, speak with your school about what kinds of events will be available to students.

Am I eligible for student health insurance?

Again, a very important question. I would bet that the answer is most likely yes. As a student, I was required to have health insurance and given the opportunity to waive the student health insurance if I opted for another plan that was comparable.

Does the school offer any sort of childcare?

Some of my classmates had young children and needed to find appropriate childcare. If your school does not offer this, they may have recommendations regarding child care centers with which they are affiliated.

Are there any options for on-campus housing?

Some students prefer to live in a dorm on-campus as this can be a convenient and cost-effective way to live. If this is something you're interested in, I suggest contacting the school sooner rather than later to discuss campus housing. On-campus housing tends to run out quickly, so if you're interested it is best to notify your school immediately upon acceptance.

Do I need a car?

Depending on where you will be living you may need a vehicle to attend classes and for transportation to your clinical sites. As I lived in Manhattan I did not need a car and was able to get anywhere I needed to go by public transportation.

What is the teacher/-student ratio?

If you're accustomed to small class settings, you may want to find out the average number of students per class. Classes can be large depending on the school and the program you're in. Some of my classes had fewer than 15 students, while others had 60.

Does the school offer job search assistance after graduation?

Although I didn't get my job through any job listings emailed to students, there were many jobs posted and sent out to students through our school of nursing list-serv. Recruiters will often contact universities with job opportunities, and your school may even hold a job fair, which may consist of a variety of organizations. This can be a great way to start your job search.

How is this program ranked nationally?

Many students like to know the national ranking of their program. If you would like to know how well ranked your potential program scores compared to others check out U.S News & World Report at http://grad-schools. usnews.rankingsandreviews.com/best-graduate-schools/top-nursing-schools/ nur-rankings.

Asking the above questions about your potential nurse practitioner program will help guide you on the path toward the school and program that best suits your needs. If possible, I recommend visiting the school and asking your questions in person with staff and students. If they have an open house that you are able to attend I suggest going as you will get a better feel for the area and may get a gut intuition if that is the right place for you. Remember not all schools are perfect and there may be parts of your program that you don't like; however, it is important to find the best fit possible and asking the above questions will help you make that decision. Now let's switch gears from deciding where you should apply to deciding which program you will actually attend.

Deciding on a Nurse Practitioner Program

Congratulations on being accepted into a nurse practitioner program! Although it may seem like you're not very far on your journey, look at where you've come from and all you have had to endure to make it to this point. Now it's time to make a decision on the best fit program for you. If you've been accepted into just one program, then the decision has already been made for you. Either you'll attend that program or wait and reapply to other programs in the future. If, on the other hand, you've received multiple acceptance letters, the decision may not be so easy.

If you're trying to decide between several programs I suggest you reread this chapter and choose which aspects of your future school are your top priorities. If you desire a school that will provide you with the least amount of debt then carefully evaluate the financial aid package being offered to you by each school. If your goal is to attend a program located in a large city, then eliminate those programs that aren't located in or near an urban environment. You get the picture; the process of elimination will help you reject programs that don't suit your needs.

As I've said earlier, a great way to help you choose a program is by actually visiting the school for yourself, and I highly suggest this if at all possible. When you're physically present at your potential school it may help you better imagine yourself as a student there or not. Many schools organize days when interested students can come by to visit such as a visiting day or an open house. This way you can actually speak with students and faculty and get the vibe of the school and neighborhood where you may be moving. If your school doesn't offer an on-campus event, you could email the office of admissions and try to set something up for yourself.

After I'd been accepted into my program, I went to "Visiting Day," which was a day held for potential students to visit the school, meet with staff and current students, and to learn and ask questions about the program. Even though I had already decided on attending Columbia, I found it incredibly helpful to participate in Visiting Day. Being on campus, surrounded by other students, solidified in my mind that I had made the right decision. That day I met people who are still my friends today and I even met my future roommate! I had a really good time touring the campus and getting to know the neighborhood where I'd spend the next several years living. I even had a bonding experience with fellow students and a security guard after being stuck in a crowded elevator (not fun but still an adventure)!

If you are still struggling to make a decision on which program to choose, I suggest writing out a pros and cons list for each school. Just the process of writing out this list may provide you with more clarity and help you reach your decision. If you still don't know what school you should attend then go with what your intuition tells you. I use my intuition daily and it never fails me; only when I ignore it am I led astray. Remember, not making a decision is still the same as making a decision. Do your best to follow your inner guidance to the program best suited for you.

As you have seen in chapter three, there are numerous types of nurse practitioner programs available to you. Deciding where to apply and then deciding where you will actually attend is a process not to be taken lightly. I wish you the best of luck making these decisions and hope you are accepted into the school of your dreams! Now that you know how the application process works and how to narrow down the programs you will be applying to, it is time to look at how you will finance your education. Chapter four is dedicated to helping you find ways to pay for your nurse practitioner education.

· 4 ·

FINANCING YOUR NURSE PRACTITIONER EDUCATION

Debt is the slavery of the free.

—Publilius Syrus

I hate to be blunt but graduate school is not cheap. Unfortunately, in this day and age there are so many students struggling with student loan debt that student loan default continues to be a widespread problem. Just applying to schools and seeing the debt you may face can be overwhelming in itself, even before you start your search for any sort of funding. When I was a student the stress of finances and debt was constantly on my mind, and on the minds of many of my classmates.

However, where there's a will there's a way and on the brighter side of things there are various ways to finance your education besides taking out a mountain of student loans and being in debt up to your ears. Returning to school is stressful enough on its own without thinking of the financial burden you must undertake. In my opinion students should be allowed to focus solely on school and not worry about how their next semester will be paid for. Sadly, this is a luxury that the majority of students don't have, and other options for financing must be sought.

This chapter will explore the variety of options available to you to finance your nurse practitioner education. As a student, I did a lot of research into financing my nurse practitioner program and have provided several of the resources (in this chapter and in the appendix) that I've used personally. Financing your graduate education can be overwhelming and I wanted to break down the resources available to you to make this part of your journey a bit less daunting.

A couple of very comprehensive resources that I suggest you take a look at are the websites www.forgetstudentloandebt.com and www.studentloan hero.com. These sites offer a ton of information available on student loan forgiveness and other means to pay for your education. Although these sites are mainly tailored to students who already have taken out loans, I suggest you check them out so you know what sort of options are available to you. Additionally, I've included in the appendix a comprehensive list of many scholarship websites and nurse practitioner organizations that offer scholarships and other financing means to help you pay for your education. Regardless if you are just starting your nurse practitioner program, are half-way through your education, or are already a practicing NP there is always financing available; you just have to know where to look. Now let's take a look at the financing options available to you, beginning with my favorite form of financing, scholarships.

Scholarships

Scholarships are free money. That's right, FREE MONEY! And who doesn't like free money?! I know that I'm a fan of it! Just a quick browse on the internet for "nursing scholarships" or "nurse practitioner scholarships" will yield a plethora of resources. It takes only a bit of research on the web to find an abundance of free money available for students in this profession.

Although scholarships are free money, some may be tied to some sort of commitment. For example, an organization may award you a scholarship only if you agree to do xyz (community service, work in an underserved community, etc.). If there is a commitment attached to the scholarship make sure you are willing and able to complete it prior to accepting the scholarship.

There are multiple scholarship websites that offer a wide variety of scholarships. Some allow you to narrow your search to specific ones applicable to you, which makes perusing the numerous scholarships much easier. Make sure you go through each scholarship carefully and eliminate those that don't apply to you. Each has its own requirements so I suggest you don't bother wasting your time applying if you don't fulfil the criteria.

There are also many scholarships that require you to write some sort of essay as part of the application. I always kept my scholarship essays as I was often able to reuse part of the essay for another scholarship as many have overlapping themes. I highly suggest you do the same; it will save you a lot of time in the future. If you are going to be applying for many scholarships it can turn into a very time-consuming process. Holding on to previous essays will help you to reduce the amount of time you spend applying.

If you're thinking, "I'll never get a scholarship because there is too much competition," you're setting yourself up for failure. Scholarships aren't just for those with a 4.0 GPA. You literally can get a scholarship for almost anything such as being the child of a veteran, your race, where you live, and even for goofy essay writing contests. I've seen scholarships you can win simply by applying without any sort of requirement, and those that were so specific I couldn't have applied even if I wanted to. I've personally received numerous scholarships simply by applying. Some I was very shocked that I received, and one I didn't even know that I had been awarded until a check showed up in the mail. I was very excited, albeit a bit confused to receive that check, but hey, free money is free money!

I'll admit that the scholarship search can be daunting. With hundreds of websites and thousands of scholarships to choose from, where do you even start your search? I recommend not trying to apply for 100 scholarships at a time as this could be very overwhelming. Narrow your search down to what is applicable to you and move from there. Prioritize deadlines and make sure you know when each scholarship is due because if you miss a deadline you will have to forfeit that scholarship.

Scholarships come in many forms and from a variety of resources. You could receive financing for one semester or for your entire education; it just depends on the parameters of the scholarship. It only takes a quick Google search to see just how much free money is available to students; a large portion of this funding is specifically designated for nurses. There are scholarships out there that would be perfect for you. You just have to do your research to find the ones that fit your eligibility and have criteria that you are able to fulfil. Several different types of scholarship options are discussed below.

Federal Government Scholarships

Although I've listed many scholarship websites in the appendix, there are a few that I wanted to write about in particular as they offer a lot of financing for nursing and nurse practitioner students. The scholarships mentioned below are funded by a branch of the government called the Health Resources and Services Administration, more commonly known as HRSA. This branch of the federal government is under the U.S. Department of Health and Human Services. One purpose of HRSA scholarships and loan repayment programs is to entice healthcare professionals to work in medically underserved communities and/or critical shortage facilities.

These scholarships come with a condition that you will work for a certain period of time to pay back what you have been awarded. Most of these scholarships require that you will spend at least two years in one of these HRSA approved medical facilities working once you graduate. However, you may be required to spend more time at a HRSA site depending on how much financing you receive. You will still be paid an NP salary; however, you will just be more limited in where you will be able to work. If you do not want to be tied to an obligation when you graduate, then I suggest you look elsewhere for financing. However, if you were already planning to work with an underserved community/population, then these scholarships may suit your needs. These scholarships can provide a lot of financing and are a great option for those who wish to minimize their debt and don't mind the commitment. The application process is quite lengthy and these scholarships are not open for application year-round. I highly advise you do your research early on to know exactly when you can apply and what you are required to submit for the application.

- Nurse Corps Scholarship Program (NCSP):
  This scholarship is allotted to nursing students who agree to commit at least two years of service to working in an underserved community. Aside from having your tuition paid for, this scholarship also allots a monthly stipend as well as money for other costs such as books and supplies. For more information visit https://bhw.hrsa.gov/loans-scholarships/nursecorps/scholarship
- National Health Service Corps (NHSC)
  This scholarship is similar to Nurse Corps but open to other health professionals as well. This is also a minimum two-year service commitment

post-graduation. You can find information on this scholarship at http://nhsc.hrsa.gov/scholarships/index.html

- Indian Health Service (IHS) Scholarship Program
This scholarship program provides scholarships to American Indian and Alaska Native students who are entering into a health profession. The scholarship provides financial support to students for a minimum two-year service commitment to an Indian health facility. Visit www.ihs.gov/scholarship for scholarship information.
- Native Hawaiian Health Scholarship (NHHS)
Similar stipulations to the other federal scholarships, but this scholarship is available only to Native Hawaiian students. The scholarship includes tuition, a monthly stipend, and other school-related costs. Recipients must work in Hawaii after receiving this award for a minimum of two years of service, depending on your award. Visit https://bhw.hrsa.gov/loansscholarships/nhhs

State-Specific Scholarships

There are many state-specific scholarships and state loan repayment programs (more on this later in the text) available for nursing and nurse practitioner students. Depending on the state, you may be eligible to apply for a variety of different funding options. Certain states offer more scholarships than others with some states offering an abundance of scholarship options. A great resource to start off with is www.nursingscholarships.org. Aside from state-specific funding, this site also discusses opportunities for other types of scholarships. I also recommend browsing the internet on state-specific nursing school scholarships. Just type in your state and include "nursing scholarship" or "nurse practitioner scholarship" and you will see that there are a ton of scholarship options out there.

Minority Student Scholarships

Minority students will find that there are many scholarships they may be eligible for. Depending on what minority category you fall under, you may have the opportunity to apply for many different scholarships, or just a few. These scholarships are scattered all over the web and, similar to other scholarships, you have to do some digging to find out which ones you are eligible to apply for. I also highly suggest that you join the nursing or NP organization of your minority (there are several listed in the appendix) as they often have scholarship opportunities available. A couple of good resources to start with are the websites www.minoritynurse.com and www.nursingscholarships.org/minority.

Nursing and Nurse Practitioner Organization Scholarships (Both State and National)

Both state and national professional nursing and nurse practitioner organizations offer scholarship opportunities (they also post jobs, too!) for nursing and nurse practitioner students. Aside from the lengthy list of scholarship websites in the appendix, there are a number of state and national nursing and NP organizations listed as well. This can be a great resource for scholarships and I highly suggest you check out this option.

Military Scholarships

Various branches of the military offer scholarships including funding for ROTC, enlisted members, and veterans. If you are interested in joining the military, or are a military veteran, these military scholarships may be just what you're looking for. Military scholarships may come directly from the military branch or from private donors. Below are a few resources for military scholarships. Again this list is not exhaustive so if you're interested in joining the military I suggest you continue looking into additional funding options and perhaps speak to a recruiter about different opportunities as well.

- US Air Force ROTC www.afrotc.com/scholarships
- Naval ROTC www.nrotc.navy.mil/scholarships.html
- Army National Guard www.nationalguard.com/tools/guard-scholarships
- US Army Health Professions Scholarship Program (HPSP) www.goarmy.com/amedd/education/hpsp.html
- www.nursingscholarships.org/military
- www.scholarships.com

Institution-Specific Scholarships

Not all funding comes from outside organizations, and there are many scholarships available that come from your academic institution. Once you're accepted into a program you may be eligible to benefit from scholarships specifically intended for students. I suggest you speak with your school's financial aid office to see what scholarships are applicable to you. Additionally, your school's alumni organization may be another great resource for institution-specific scholarships. Often you are eligible for more than one scholarship at a time.

Another resource that offers school-based loans and scholarships is HRSA. Check out the website at https://bhw.hrsa.gov/loansscholarships/schoolbasedloans; it offers several options for students including multiple student loan options. Your school must participate in the program in order for you to be eligible to apply.

Disability Scholarships

A great resource for scholarships as well as resources for nurses and nursing students with disabilities is www.exceptionalnurse.com. There are several scholarships available to apply for on this site.

Gender-Based Scholarships

There are scholarships available specifically for men in nursing and for women in nursing. The American Association for Men in Nursing offers several scholarships on their website specifically for male nurses. Visit www.aamn.org for more information.

There is an entire website dedicated to scholarships for women found at www.scholarshipsforwomen.net. You can also check out the Jeannette Rankin Women's Scholarship Fund at www.rankinfoundation.org.

LGBTQ Scholarships

You can also apply to scholarships as an LGBTQ student. Below is a list of the websites that offer many scholarships and resources for those who identify as LGBTQ.

- www.pointfoundation.org
- www.gammamufoundation.org
- www.pridefoundation.org
- www.equityfoundation.org
- www.campuspride.org
- www.pflag.org

Other Scholarship Resources

There are many other options for scholarships aside from those listed above. Other places to consider looking for funding include but are not limited to small and large businesses, religious organizations, and private donors.

Grants

Grants, similar to scholarships, are free money, and as I asked before, who doesn't like free money? Many grants are awarded on a need basis, which is your financial status, instead of a merit basis, which is more applicable to scholarships. Grants can also be awarded for projects, such as research projects, and are not necessarily available just for students but for those in the workforce as well.

Funding for grants can come from multiple resources such as state government, federal government, private sector, and nonprofit organizations. To be eligible for federal grants as well as other federal financial aid resources visit www.fafsa.ed.gov. You will have to fill out the financial aid form to be eligible for certain grants. There will be more information on FAFSA below in the student loan section. Another resource for grants can be found at https://studentaid.ed.gov/sa/types/grants-scholarships.

Student Loan Repayment Programs

Now that we've covered scholarships and grants let's talk about student loan repayment programs. This is another very popular option among students and former students to have part or all of their loans paid off, usually in exchange for working in an underserved community, which I mentioned above. The type of facility you will be required to work in depends on the program under which you receive the award. Loan repayment programs differ from scholarships and grants as the former are free money, and with loan repayment programs you actually have to borrow the money up front, and then apply to a program to have it paid back.

The thing to remember about student loan repayment programs is that you typically have to have the job first prior to applying to a program. Loan repayment is also not guaranteed and vying for these coveted spots can be fierce. I suggest checking out several different loan repayment programs as different programs have different stipulations and you'll need to determine which program best suits your need. The amount of financing awarded also varies by program. Below a variety of loan repayment options are discussed.

Federal Loan Repayment Programs

The federal government offers several different options for students to repay their loans by working in medically underserved communities, which are given numerical scores. The higher the score the more underserved the site. Loan repayment programs help alleviate the student loan debt burden and also place healthcare professionals in areas that are medically underserved. It is important to note that federal loan repayment is not guaranteed for everyone and competition can be intense.

If you are interested in a federal loan repayment program, make sure to do your research prior to accepting a job to ensure it is a qualified site. Just because you think an area is medically underserved doesn't mean that the government has deemed it to be. Site-specific information can be found online, and if you still have additional questions, you can contact the loan repayment agency for verification.

The application process can be arduous so I suggest getting all documents together early. Unfortunately, due to the high volume of applicants, you may have to wait months before you even hear if you have been accepted into the program. Once you've been offered an award make sure you will be able to fulfill the requirements prior to accepting it. If you don't think you can fulfill the commitment such as working forty hours a week for two years, then I suggest you look for other sources of funding. If you default on a federal student loan repayment program, this could mean repaying everything back plus interest.

As you will see from the list below, there are several different federal loan repayment programs available. I know several people who have received loan repayment through these government programs, and they can be incredibly lucrative. I also have a friend who applied one year and didn't receive funding but reapplied the next year and got the award. An NP colleague of mine even received federal loan repayment as well as state loan repayment (discussed next) at the same time. Talk about hitting the jackpot! Now let's take a look at several options available for loan repayment.

- National Health Service Corps (NHSC) Loan Repayment Program. You can apply for this program once you've graduated and found a job at a qualified site. Loan repayment can be a substantial amount and this is a very popular option among NP graduates. For more information visit https://nhsc.hrsa.gov/loanrepayment/loanrepaymentprogram.html
- Nurse Corps Loan Repayment Program. This program offers loan forgiveness of up to 85% of your debt. You can find more information about this program at https://bhw.hrsa.gov/loansscholarships/nurse-corps/lrp.
- Indian Health Service Loan Repayment Program. This federal loan repayment program offers up to $40,000 in loan repayment (on top of your regular NP salary) for a two-year commitment at a qualifying site that serves Alaska Native and American Indian communities. More information on this loan repayment program can be found at https://www.ihs.gov/loanrepayment.
- Faculty Loan Repayment. You can receive loan repayment if you are interested in a career as faculty at a "health professions school." With this loan repayment option you can receive up to $40,000 in assistance. For more information you can visit https://bhw.hrsa.gov/loans scholarships/flrp.

State Loan Repayment Programs (SLRP)

Individual states also offer incentives such as state loan repayment for nurses and nurse practitioners. States have their own individual programs, but many are similar to the federal government programs that incentivize health providers to work in medically underserved communities. Some states offer greater repayment than others, and some states offer more than one program. You can find state-specific state loan repayment programs with a quick Google search. I've also included some state loan repayment options in the appendix.

Military College Loan Repayment Program

This student loan repayment program is available to those who have already accumulated student loans and who decide to join the military. Each military branch offers different incentives and has different criteria, so it's important to find out which loans will be forgiven prior to enlisting. Again, a quick Google search will help you find the resources available to best suit your needs.

Public Service Loan Forgiveness

The Public Service Loan Forgiveness (PSLF) program is another way to reduce your debt burden. This program is not available to everyone, but is for those who have been working for a qualifying employer—such as for the government or nonprofit organization. If you qualify, the PSLF program will forgive the remainder of your direct loans after you have made 120 "qualifying" payments on your loans. This must be done while working full-time for a qualifying employer. For more information check out https://studentaid.ed.gov/sa/repay-loans/forgiveness-cancellation/public-service.

Teaching Assistant (TA)

Many schools offer the opportunity for students to work as a teaching assistant in exchange for tuition credit. In general, a TA helps the professor with class tasks such as responding to student emails, facilitating study groups, managing online content, and whatever else the professor may need. For example, if you are a TA in a three-credit class, you may be eligible to receive up to three credits in free tuition. The amount you receive obviously depends on your school, so make sure to get specifics before you decide to commit to a position.

If you have extra time to work as a TA, this can be a great way to pay for tuition as costs really add up. I was a TA myself and I'm very grateful to have had this opportunity to help finance my education as it significantly reduced my debt burden. If you are interested in this option you can contact your school's Office of Financial Aid to get information on how to become a TA. Usually you must have taken the class prior to being a TA for that course. An added benefit of being a TA is that it's a great refresher course to relearn material that you may have forgotten.

Tip. If you're going to be a TA make sure you organize yourself accordingly. As a TA, you are also a student and may concomitantly be working. It's imperative that you allot yourself enough time to complete your TA duties. You are usually the go-to for student questions so make sure any information you are relaying is clear and succinct. Otherwise you may be bombarded with loads of time-consuming questions. You will also most likely get many emails from students so remember to be patient with them and answer in a timely fashion, just as you'd expect from a TA in one of your classes.

Student Loans

Student loans are used by a majority of students to help finance their education. However, I deliberately put this section at the end as I highly recommend seeking other sources of financing such as scholarships and grants before taking out a mountain of student loans. I am by no means an expert on student loans (although I've taken out a good portion of them); however, I wanted to highlight the differences between loans so you can get a better sense of which option is best for you. I suggest you speak to your school's financial aid office about the specifics if you have questions on loans. They are a great resource and their job is to help students fund their education.

Prior to taking out government loans you will need to fill out the free application for federal student aid (FAFSA). This will be sent to your school and helps to determine your financial aid package. More information on the FAFSA can be found at www.fafsa.gov. Essentially, you have two options when taking out loans: federal loans and private loans. Federal loans are loans borrowed from the federal government. It is definitely recommended that you begin your borrowing with federal loans over private loans as they are most likely lower in interest and have certain perks that private loans do not have. Private loans are often used to supplement tuition and living expenses once federal loans have been maxed out. These are usually given by banks or private lending institutions. For more information on federal versus private loans visit https://studentaid.ed.gov/sa/types/loans/federal-vs-private

———

As you have seen in this chapter there are a number of ways to finance your nurse practitioner education. From free money in the form of scholarships and grants to student loan repayment programs, there is an abundance of financing options available. While doing my research for this chapter I was astounded at just how many scholarships are available to nursing students. I definitely think it's worth your time and effort to spend time looking for and applying to scholarships as you may be able to finance your entire education without taking out a single student loan! If you've already graduated and are reading this chapter, then definitely look into the loan repayment options discussed. Although the search for free money and loan repayment programs may seem cumbersome, your future self will thank you!

· 5 ·

GETTING THROUGH YOUR NURSE PRACTITIONER PROGRAM

I attribute my success to this—I never gave or took any excuse.

—Florence Nightingale

Congratulations, you have come a long way on your journey to becoming a nurse practitioner! After months, or perhaps years, of completing prerequisite courses, applying to numerous nurse practitioner programs, and searching for financing for your education, you are finally ready to begin your nurse practitioner program. This is an exciting yet scary time as you will be journeying into new and unfamiliar territory.

For some of you it will be a completely new field, having never worked in healthcare before. You may be wondering what exactly is in store for you, perhaps never having been in a clinical setting in your life. For others, maybe you have been working as an RN for years and have decided to return to school to further your career. You could be feeling a mixture of excitement coupled with anxiety about returning to the academic world. Regardless of where you are in life, if you have just entered into the field or have been a nurse for years, the role of the nurse practitioner is quite different than that of a registered nurse and you may go through some life adjustments preparing for this new responsibility.

I've heard people naysay new nurses going directly into a nurse practitioner program after having recently completed their BSN without having any previous RN experience first. Some believe that NP students should have at least a year (or more) of RN floor experience prior to pursuing advanced studies. While any kind of nursing experience will help you in the clinical setting, as stated above, an RN and an NP function in two completely different roles. If someone tells you that you need more nursing experience in order to become a great nurse practitioner, kindly smile and thank them for their advice and continue on your way. Hard work, dedication, and always doing what's best for your patients will make you the great nurse practitioner you want to be, not just your previous nursing experience.

Nurse Practitioner Program Basics

This chapter is designed to help you successfully get through and complete your nurse practitioner program. Regardless of what specialty you are pursuing or what school you attend, this chapter will help set you up for success. Even though the information in this chapter is aimed to be a guide, I can't get into specific details since each to program varies tremendously. Nevertheless, the general content of this chapter is applicable to a wide range of programs and specialties. Despite the fact that each individual nurse practitioner program is structured differently, they must meet certain requirements to be accredited by the Commission on Collegiate Nursing Education (CCNE).

Now, let's get into some of the good stuff and take a look at the general structure of your nurse practitioner program.

Orientation

You will most likely have a required orientation prior to starting your program. Orientation is designed to do just that, to orient you to your new program and school. During this time, you will have an opportunity to review your program plan, meet fellow students and faculty, and get to know the school better. You may be given a tour of the facilities such as the campus, library, offices, and gym if available. Orientation gives you the opportunity to ask questions and address concerns you may have about your upcoming program.

During your orientation, you may be informed of what is expected of you as a student, such as maintaining a certain GPA. You will also be informed of what will happen if you do not meet those requirements. Orientation is a very important part of your overall experience to beginning your NP program. Not only will you get to know other students and staff, but it will also help to clear up any confusion you may have. I suggest paying attention and taking notes. If orientation is not required, it is highly recommended that you attend. The information presented during your orientation is exceptionally valuable and may answer many of your questions or help calm your fears. You may even meet your new best friend!

Didactic Courses

Prior to starting your clinical rotations, or perhaps taken concomitantly while in clinical, you will be completing didactic courses, which are held in the class-room. Didactic courses cover a wide variety of nursing-related topics. I cannot generalize too much here as each specialty will have different requirements and every program is structured differently. However, some of the courses you may be taking may include pharmacology, diagnosis and management, nursing theory, healthcare policies, as well as a variety of science and nursing courses. Your pro-gram plan should indicate clearly which classes you will be required to complete.

During this classroom time, you will be given an enormous amount of content to learn. Didactic courses can be challenging as it will seem like you have to learn everything in a very short amount of time. It's in your best inter-est to use this time wisely. Ask questions, discuss cases with professors and fellow students, and soak up as much knowledge as you can. You will soon be putting what you have learned to practical use.

Time Management

It is imperative to balance your time wisely in NP school. Many things are being thrown at you throughout your studies, and time management is essen-tial to your success. I found it very helpful to have a paper planner with me at all times to help me manage my time. I started by using the calendar on my phone, but this was confusing as I was constantly adding and crossing off assignments and making changes to my schedule. I then tried using both the calendar on my phone and a planner; however, this confused me even more as sometimes I would forget to put a date in one—thus both had different schedules. I finally ended up sticking with just my paper planner as this allowed me to visualize in front of me everything that I had to do for the upcoming day and week. It was also extremely satisfying to check off something that I had completed. Many of my classmates also lived with their planner always at their side, to make sure they jotted down important due dates or last-minute notes. To this day I continue to use a paper planner, which has allowed me to be much more organized with my daily life.

While I was in NP school I often used the time/benefit analysis to decide if I should undertake an activity as my time was incredibly valuable. Since I lived in Manhattan I was able to drop laundry off at virtually any laundromat to have it washed, dried, and folded. Although this service costs more than washing and drying the clothes myself, the time that I saved paying for this laundry service was in my opinion more beneficial than saving the money by doing it myself. I often used those extra two or three hours to study and was always grateful for this opportunity.

Each person manages his or her time differently and it is important to know how you function in order to maximize your time most efficiently. For example, if you know you are a procrastinator and work best under pressure, don't schedule yourself for a 12-hour work shift the night before an important assignment is due. On the other hand, if you don't like to procrastinate and like to get things done once they are assigned, make sure you have enough time allotted to complete the assignment. I don't do well under pressure for assignments so I'd actually start the assignment soon after it was assigned to ensure I had a game plan and enough time to complete it.

Time management also saved my life while I was both working and in school. Some days were just insane as I would start my job around eight or nine in the morning, then around midday I would have class for two to three hours (thankfully on the same campus), and then I'd get on the subway and take the 45-minute commute to clinical where I would stay until midnight. After a long day of work, class, and clinical I would often not get home until after one o'clock in the morning. I sure don't miss those days as they were brutal and I had to effectively manage my time (and my sanity) to get through them.

Books and Office Supplies

I've often been asked the question about what books were helpful during life as a student. Since professors require or suggest multiple readings or texts, buying books can become incredibly expensive. My first year in nursing school

I bought several books brand new. Realizing that there were cheaper options, I then would rent books or buy them used online or from other students. I eventually realized that I wasn't using the books I had purchased after the class was finished, and so I stopped spending money on them altogether. For me, this was the best solution as I didn't want to keep accumulating books that I wouldn't read. Additionally, there are so many great online resources that are far more convenient. Nevertheless, there were certain texts that I became familiar with and would use over and over again (especially in clinical). I became judicious in what I purchased as I wanted resources that I would use not only as a student but also as a practicing NP.

I am very grateful that throughout my time as an NP student, I had easy access to computers, scanners, and printers. I was constantly scanning documents and printing out lectures, health documents, reports, and papers at the university library. Both a scanner and printer were crucial to me, and if your school does not provide these items I suggest purchasing them yourself.

I also recommend investing in a quality laptop computer for your time as a student. My laptop was invaluable to me and I used it for everything from writing papers to binge watching Netflix when I needed a break. I always had my MacBook Air with me to take notes and to reference material during the lecture. This computer saved my life as it is lightweight and powers on immediately when it is opened. Not that I am promoting Mac over other brands, it's just that this computer fits my needs and I couldn't have survived NP school without it. I suggest researching laptops prior to starting your program to ensure you have the best fit for you.

Studying Pearls

Studying will be a very large component of your NP program and isn't to be taken lightly. I spent a large portion of my program at the library, and did very well because of it. Although I've met several students who rarely opened a book except to prepare for an upcoming exam, I don't recommend this strategy unless you are a genius! Throughout your program you will be bombarded with knowledge from all different sources on dozens of subjects. It is impossible to remember all this information! Reviewing your notes from a previous lecture or studying the PowerPoints and resources given out by your instructors can be very beneficial. Additionally, now that I am in clinical practice I still use the resources provided for me during my time as a student. I recommend holding on to the resources you find helpful as you never know when you'll need to use them again.

Each person studies differently and it is by no means my place to tell you how best to study. However, I do recommend finding a place to study that works for you and sticking with it. Some people need background noise to study, so a coffee shop may be a good option for you. For others, myself included, a nice quiet area is the only way I can concentrate so I work best in the library or in an area free of noise. Knowing your study habits will help you study more efficiently and be more effective with your time.

Although your life consists of many facets beyond the books, you went to NP school for a reason, so make it a priority to study. You don't want to get to the point where you haven't done so hot in a few classes and now you're on academic probation. I had a lot of fun throughout my NP program years; however, I made studying a priority and usually waited until I was done for the day to let loose and unwind. I suggest you incorporate studying into your calendar the same as you'd do for your gym class; write it down and stick to it. I planned my weekends around my study habits, and I knew that I couldn't really unwind that night until I'd accomplished what I thought was a satisfactory amount of studying.

Below I've listed several study tips I have used that may help you with your studies. Use what applies to you and leave the rest. We all learn differently but I wanted to offer what has worked for me as this may help you as well.

Attend Lectures

I can't emphasize enough how important it is to consistently attend your lectures. Yes, we have all missed a class or two for various reasons; however, I suggest not making this a habit. Aside from covering required material, lectures are also very important as professors will often present material in person that was not on PowerPoint lectures. They may also use their own clinical experiences and anecdotes to relay information about the topic. I found some of my most helpful lectures were those when a professor directly related the information presented in class to a clinical scenario. Your professors may point out important concepts that you will be tested on that are not located in your readings. Also, attending class may be a requirement and you may have to sign in to verify your attendance. If you are not there you may get points deducted, which is another reason to attend class!

Pay Attention in Class

This may seem like a no-brainer, but trust me, four-hour lectures can become very tedious and it may be difficult to give the material your undivided attention. I always brought my computer to lecture so I had the opportunity to browse the internet. Although it brought a welcome relief when I was beginning to crash from all the information, if I wasn't careful I would end up on it for longer than intended, often missing key points. Hopefully if your classes are this long you will be given breaks to stretch and recharge your brain. However, if not, I recommend getting up and stretching once in a while to keep focused on the material.

Take Notes

Throughout my time as a nurse practitioner student I would vacillate between taking detailed notes and not taking very good notes. I've noticed that some students prefer to sit and listen, absorbing all the information without ever having to jot anything down. Others would print out all the lecture material and meticulously write out whatever the professor was saying. Regardless if you are a note taker or not, always have something on hand to jot an important fact down. I don't know how many times randomly throughout the lecture a teacher would say, "Study this, it may be on the exam." We'd all be scrambling to write that information down as we would be tested on it sooner or later.

Flashcards

These are a great way to study and learn material. Just the act of writing things down reinforces them in your brain. Flashcards are a great way to study, especially if you're on the go. I used these to study while riding the subway, which really helped me supplement my learning. I also used flashcards to study with friends as we were able to quiz one another. There are several websites that allow you to make your own flashcards for free such as www.quizlet.com. You can also make flashcards on the go for your smartphone at sites such as www.cram.com.

Videos

Videos offer an excellent opportunity to supplement your learning. You can sit back, relax, and just learn. If you're tired of reading textbooks and lecture PowerPoints, try watching a video. While in school I found that YouTube videos were a great way to complement my learning. If I didn't understand a concept (which was often the case) I would watch YouTube videos over and over again until I really comprehended the material. If you are a visual learner this may be a great way for you to learn concepts as you are actually visualizing what is happening. This was most helpful for me when learning the anatomy of organ systems, especially the blood circulation of the heart. These videos were also helpful when I was preparing for my board examination.

Study Groups

Study groups are a great way to connect with other students while learning and working through challenging material and concepts together. If you find you learn well in a group setting, I highly suggest you find other students who have similar study habits and partner up with them. I recommend studying the material individually prior to a study group session as you may be lost once you enter the group if you're not up to date on the concepts. I found that my learning increased exponentially while participating in study groups. My classmates were able to explain material to me that I didn't understand, and we were able to work through difficult concepts together. I'd also learn study tips, acronyms, and other helpful hints from my fellow classmates. We'd all hunker down in a sterile room in the library for hours—drawing images on the whiteboard, chatting, and of course eating food ordered from Grubhub. There is also something comforting about being with others while studying for hours in the middle of the night.

Review Sessions

While I was a student, often a professor or teaching assistant would hold a review session prior to an upcoming exam. These sessions were incredibly helpful as they helped guide our studying and would also clarify questions we had on subject material. Instructors may also review the breakdown of content on the exam, something that is very useful to know. If your professor offers a review session I encourage you to attend as this is a very helpful way to review key concepts before the test. If this is not usually done at your school, try asking your professor if this can be arranged.

Other Study Resources

Aside from going to class and studying, there are a million resources out there to help supplement your education. If you would like to learn more about a subject covered in class or expand your knowledge, I encourage you to seek out these opportunities. My university and local teaching hospital always offered lectures, grand rounds, guest speakers, continuing education conferences, and other seminars to keep staff and students informed and educated.

The Clinical Experience

Now that we've covered what the didactic part of your program will be like, let's talk about clinical. Throughout this book I've mentioned "clinical" several times in reference to the clinical portion of your NP program. However, you may still be wondering what exactly clinical entails. Thus, I've dedicated the next part of this book to explaining clinical and what you will be doing during this time. Now, let's get into the nitty gritty about clinical!

So, What Exactly Is Clinical?

Clinical is the student experience you have in a clinical setting that takes place outside of the classroom. You will need to complete a certain number of clinical hours prior to graduation. Your time in clinical will be spent at a designated location(s), usually chosen by your program. However, you may also have the option available to choose your own clinical site if your program director agrees. Essentially, your clinical hours can be in virtually any healthcare setting that is within the scope of practice within your NP specialty. In chapter one, I listed many different areas where NPs work. I suggest you reference this to get a better understanding of where you may be placed while in clinical.

As a nurse practitioner student, I was placed in several different clinical settings working with a variety of preceptors. This was very helpful as I was able to learn how different clinics were managed and how the clinic flow affected the day. I felt I fit in better at some sites than others, but I always learned something valuable from every clinical placement. I also learned an incredible amount with each provider and preceptor I worked with. Not that I necessarily agreed with how they practiced all the time, but it was good for me to also see what I didn't consider good medicine. Even after you've completed your studies and are a practicing NP you will continuously be learning from each setting that you work in, and from the different healthcare providers who will now be your colleagues.

Starting off your clinical rotations as an NP student can be daunting. As mentioned before, the function of an NP is completely different from that of an RN. Be easy with yourself as this role can take some getting used to. Be patient as you will make mistakes and feel inept from time to time. This is all part of the journey to becoming the amazing nurse practitioner that you desire to be. Having a great clinical experience can really help boost your confidence as a student. This is the time where you will really see how NPs function and you'll gain a deeper understanding about medicine, nursing, and the patients you treat.

As an NP student, I was placed at several different clinical sites. One of my favorite clinical rotations was at a pediatric urgent care, which helped develop my love for both pediatrics and urgent care. I learned a great deal from all of the pediatricians with whom I worked, and I still use the knowledge that I learned there in my current clinical practice. Another site was at an adult outpatient clinic with a large West African population as this is where the doctor was from. This was a similar patient population, to my Peace Corps days, and I loved the culture and interacting with the patients. As you can see, both of these patient populations are completely different from one another; however, I still was able to learn a great deal from each site.

Clinical Uniforms and Supplies

Depending on your program and your clinical location you will most likely be wearing scrubs or business casual apparel with or without a white coat during your clinical rotations. I wore scrubs throughout my BSN clinical rotations and then a white coat with business casual attire during the master's portion. Your attire may change depending on where you are placed.

If you are required to wear scrubs many institutions have standard scrub uniforms. If you are allowed a bit of creativity in your uniform good for you, just keep it professional. There are many websites where you can buy affordable scrubs, and you may also be able to buy used scrubs from graduating students. This will bring the price down significantly and the scrubs can still be in pretty good condition.

As far as clinical supplies to purchase, your school will most likely give you a list of what you need. My school gave me a list of supplies and I purchased all of the required items. However, I ended up not needing or using them all. Many sites have supplies on hand but sometimes I would bring my own such as a reflex hammer or penlight. The one thing that I could not live without is my stethoscope, which I took with me everywhere. A good quality stethoscope can go a long way, and I suggest not skimping on this purchase.

Preceptors

I've mentioned preceptors several times throughout the text, so now let's get into what a preceptor actually is and the role they perform. While you are completing your clinical hours, you will be supervised and mentored by a preceptor. A preceptor is someone who is designated to help you develop your clinical skills. Their job is to teach you how to implement all the classroom knowledge you've learned into the clinical setting.

While in clinical you most likely will have several different people who will precept you. Preceptors for nurse practitioner students can range from seasoned NPs to new graduate NPs, to physicians. You will learn from each preceptor as each provider has their own style of practicing and will offer a different insight into patient care. Preceptor arrangements come in many forms. For example, you may shadow your preceptor while they see their patients or you may see the patient first and then present to the preceptor after. Or, you both may enter the patient room at the same time and you will watch the interaction between preceptor and patient. It just depends on the preceptor's preferences as well as your clinical skills and confidence level.

While you are under the guidance of a preceptor you will have the opportunity to ask questions in a safe and nonjudgmental setting. This is the time to learn as much as you can as soon you will be on your own. Having a great preceptor can make for a great clinical experience and you may even develop a long-standing relationship with this person. I still speak with some of my preceptors and I am incredibly grateful for all the knowledge they instilled in me.

How to Find a Preceptor

Some programs find preceptor placements for their students while other programs require you to find your own preceptor. If your program does not place you with a clinical preceptor, then it is your duty to go out and find someone to precept you. If you already have a preceptor or you will be placed by your program, you may still want to read this section as students who already have preceptor placements often look for other preceptors in different facilities.

Depending on your circumstances it may be relatively easy to find a preceptor, or it may require a bit of effort on your part. I recommend starting with the contacts you already have within your geographic area. You could begin by asking around and inquiring of your classmates if they know of anyone who would be able to precept you. If you are working as an RN in a clinical setting that is within your NP scope of practice, you can ask some of your provider colleagues if they'd be willing to precept you. This is how some of my friends found preceptors; they just asked their work colleagues. Your local NP association may also be a resource to help you find someone who is willing to precept you. Additionally, if there is a certain person you'd like to learn from, go ahead and reach out to them. You never know who will say yes, so I suggest asking anyone with whom you would like to work. Some health professionals love to precept and teach students while others do not and feel like students are a hindrance. I suggest finding the former and avoiding the latter!

While finding a preceptor you want to avoid settings that treat you as an employee and not a student. I've had classmates find themselves in an uncomfortable position as they were relied upon to see patients while they were students and found themselves in awkward situations when they couldn't attend clinical on certain days. Remember you are a student, and if a clinical site treats you as an employee I suggest you speak with whomever is in charge of your clinical placement about this.

Preceptor Advice

- You are there to learn. Remember that it's the preceptor's job to teach you as you are the student. Although the majority of preceptors are not paid, their job is to be a good mentor and teacher. If you do not find you are learning enough from the person you were placed with, you can ask for someone new.

- Be respectful. This may seem like a no-brainer but I've heard many stories of my classmates disagreeing with how the preceptor managed a patient and letting their preceptor know they were wrong. Remember, each provider practices differently and, even though we may not agree with what they are doing, this is also a good teaching tool as we learn not only what we should do, but also what we should not.
- Be punctual, if not early. Wherever you are doing your clinical rotation you are most likely going to hit the ground running. Getting to your site early may help you feel a bit more prepared for the day ahead of you. You can orient yourself to the schedule for that day and see what types of patients you will be seeing. Being punctual also shows your professionalism and makes you look better.
- Dress professionally. Arriving at clinical dressed as a professional and not just a student is a good way to practice being in the real world. Would you want to go see a sloppily dressed healthcare provider?
- Always thank your preceptor at the end of your clinical time together. This can also be done throughout your clinical rotation, but especially at the end. I usually gave preceptors a handwritten note and/ or a small gift to show my appreciation. A gift is not required or expected, but a handwritten note can go a long way. Remember this individual has spent many hours working with you and teaching you, so it's important to acknowledge and be grateful for all that you've learned from them.

From Student Clinician to Employee

Keep in the back of your mind that many clinical placements can lead to jobs once you graduate and are a board certified and licensed NP. Although I advise that you perform your best whether you are interested in a job there or not, this is especially true if you'd like to turn your clinical experience into a future paid position. If you would like to work at your facility once you graduate, make sure you learn how things work in the clinic. This includes the electronic medical record (EMR), clinical flow, how to order lab tests and imaging, how to refer patients to specialists, and where medicines and supplies are kept. This will make your transition from student to clinician so much easier and quicker for you.

While I was completing my doctorate, my very last clinical placement turned into a paid position. The transition from student to employee was relatively easy and took off a lot of the "new job jitters" that can be quite daunting, especially in a new field. I already knew how the clinic functioned and was comfortable working with the staff. It was a great experience for me, too, as it was a clinic run by NPs. How amazing! If your potential employer sees that you can hit the ground running once you are in a paid position, the argument to hire you is that much stronger!

Getting Involved in Your School

So far in this chapter we've covered just about everything you need to know regarding life as an NP student. However, we haven't talked about on-campus activities that are not affiliated with your NP program. As a former nurse practitioner student, I can personally attest to the hectic life you will be trying to balance. Between studying, classes, clinical, and possibly working, at times your life may be fully scheduled from sunrise to way past sundown. Nevertheless, I encourage you to stay connected with your school and community as this will help to enrich your nurse practitioner student experience.

There may be an Office of Student Services (or another similarly titled department) at your school that organizes events for students. If there is, I recommend checking in with them to see what services and events they provide for their students. My school of nursing would send out a weekly email of the social functions happening that week with information about upcoming future events as well. They sponsored a ton of cool events from dances to craft events to yoga classes that were available exclusively to students. Although my schedule didn't permit me to participate in a lot of these events, the ones that I did attend I found very enjoyable, and it was fun to socialize with my peers outside of the classroom.

Aside from social event planning, the Office of Student Services would also email information on upcoming volunteer positions for local health fairs and community events that both nursing and NP students could participate in. At these health fairs we'd take blood pressures, check glucose and lipid levels, and discuss healthy lifestyles with the people who attended. I really enjoyed participating in these events as I learned new clinical skills and it was a great way to be of service and get to know the community. These volunteer activities can be really great experiences, and if you have the opportunity to participate I encourage that you do. You will not only be providing valuable services, but you will also be improving your clinical skills.

As a student, I also had the opportunity to attend a Nurse Practitioner Lobby Day which was put on by the state NP association. This was an incredible experience where several of my classmates and I traveled to the capital for an overnight trip. We had the privilege to meet with other amazing NPs from around the state lobbying for several laws. That day was very interesting to me as it was the first time I heard NPs talk in a political sense. Being there made me excited about the future and I felt especially proud to be part of such an amazing profession. Being involved with your school may lead you to similar experiences, so stay connected!

It also helps to stay in the loop by getting to know the staff at your school. From helping you out with financial aid to organizing social events, the staff at your school can be a great resource, and they are the true heroes behind the scenes. As an NP student, I had the opportunity to get to know a lot of the staff who were incredibly wonderful people. They always asked how I was doing and helped me out every step of the way. If your school staff is as supportive as mine was, you will definitely have no trouble staying involved and feeling supported by your school.

Getting involved as a student may also help you find a job once you graduate. Many schools organize job fairs or career days where they invite companies to the school to provide information about their organization. This can be a great way to meet potential future employers and really get a feel for what the NP job market is like. While I was a student, I attended events in which both potential employers and residency programs participated. They provided a great deal of information about their organizations and students were able to ask questions and gain more insight as to what each organization was all about.

Enjoy Yourself

As you can see from the previous pages in this chapter, getting through and surviving your nurse practitioner program is much more than just going to class. There are your clinical obligations, classroom requirements, hours and hours of studying, and of course your multiple examinations. In addition to your school commitments, you may also be working a full- or part-time job. You may also have a family, and between all of your obligations may not get a moment to yourself. Nevertheless, it is important to find balance in all these things that you do and I highly recommend that you enjoy the ride.

When I first started my BSN program I was very focused on studying and would only go out once everything was completed. I'd often find myself stressing about upcoming classes and deadlines even when I was out with friends. Trust me, it's no fun to be out on the town in Manhattan only to find yourself worrying about an upcoming exam! However, over time, once I became more accustomed to the rigor of the program, I was able to relax with the firm belief that I would not fail out of NP school, and I began to enjoy myself more. I finally realized that I was going to become a nurse practitioner regardless of what I did during my free time and I might as well enjoy myself during the process.

When I was a Peace Corps Volunteer I used to have a hanging wall calendar where I'd write something to look forward to each month. This may also help you during NP school so you can actually visualize something fun coming up. Maybe it's a birthday party for a friend or a play you really want to see. Regardless of how small the event may be, write it down and stick to it. You are going to burn yourself out if you don't bring a little lightness into your student life.

Being a student can and will be incredibly overwhelming at times. Remember, "this too shall pass" and nothing, not even the stress of an upcoming exam, will last forever. Try to make the most out of your NP student experience. Go out with friends, take a day off from studying, exercise! Keep yourself in a good place mentally, physically, and emotionally and just enjoy being a student.

———

I hope that this chapter gave you more clarity and insight on how to survive and excel in your nurse practitioner program. We've covered a multitude of topics to help prepare you for what is to come, and hopefully you'll be feeling a bit more at ease with the next phase of your NP journey. Now that you are more familiar with the process, it's time to switch gears as you transition from graduation to beginning your practice as an NP.

· 6 ·

AFTER GRADUATION, NOW WHAT?

Whatever you decide to do, make sure it makes you happy.

—Paulo Coelho

Throughout the previous chapters you've had a chance to understand what a nurse practitioner is and does, as well as get a better feeling for the diversity of the field. We've covered everything from the role of a nurse practitioner to how to get accepted into a program and successfully complete your nurse practitioner program. Although you most likely have learned a lot about how to proceed after you graduate, there are still many things that can be confusing when making the transition from student to clinician.

Though you may be ready for a break after completing your rigorous studies, there are several steps that need to be taken between graduation and actually starting off your practice as an NP. When I was a new graduate, there was a lot of confusion surrounding everything that needed to be done prior to actually starting my first job. There was much that I had to learn the hard and long way, and I thought it best to walk you through the steps that need to be taken to become a practicing nurse practitioner.

Board Certification

To legally practice in the majority of states you need to be board certified. Board certification is a professional recognition you will be eligible for after you've finished your nurse practitioner education at an accredited institution. To become board certified you need to successfully pass the national examination in your specialty.

I recommend taking your board certifying examination as soon as possible after you graduate as the material will still be fresh in your head. Aside from this, there is also your future job to consider. As you will need to be board certified in order to work as a nurse practitioner, you would hate to find yourself in the position of having a job offer but not being able to start as you haven't yet taken your boards.

Several different organizations offer board certification exams for nurse practitioners. The certifying body will depend on the specialty or subspecialty under which you wish to be certified. I do not recommend one certifying body over another; each organization is different and it is important to evaluate which one will best fit your needs. Certain certifying bodies will offer discounts on national certification if you are already a member or student member with their organization. To help with your research I've listed a variety of different board certifying organizations in the appendix.

It is important to remember that if you would like to be board certified in a subspecialty such as dermatology, you must first be board certified in your primary specialty (family, adult, etc.). Make sure you research the exact requirements you need if you are planning on getting board certified in a subspecialty. The educational requirements should have been fulfilled during the subspecialty component of your program; however, it is up to you to do your due diligence to ensure everything is in order prior to taking the test.

Preparing for and sitting for your board examination can be a stressful experience. Yet it is important to remember that your nurse practitioner program should have adequately prepared you for successful completion of the examination (coupled with a lot of additional studying on your part). Just think of it as another standardized test, one of many that you have already completed. Don't psych yourself out too much. Most likely you will pass on the first try, and if not you will just need to retake the exam.

Studying for Your Board Examination

The day before I was to sit for my family nurse practitioner board examination was a complete nightmare. Looking back on that time I can't believe that I actually passed my boards. I arrived back in New York City with my father whom I had flown to Michigan to see the previous week. His health was declining and his doctors couldn't figure out why, so I flew to Michigan and brought him back with me to be seen at my university's hospital. He had a doctor's appointment at the hospital a few hours after we landed. Once he'd been seen at his office visit, the physician recommended we take him to the emergency room as it was the quickest way he would be able to be admitted into the hospital. I remember sitting with him in the emergency room waiting to see where this journey would lead, not knowing that he would pass away within six weeks. After a long day of travel from Michigan to NYC, a doctor's appointment, and now an emergency room visit, I finally had to say goodbye as my board exam was early the next morning.

On the subway ride to the testing center I pumped myself up with "All Right Now" by Free, trying to psych myself up. Even though the previous week was terrible, I had studied for months prior to that and had to have faith that I would pass, which I did. Looking back at that unbelievably tough time I sometimes wonder how I passed with so much personal stress in my life. I think it was sheer determination and adequate preparation that helped me get through that test.

Now I'm guessing that your board examination probably won't be as stressful as mine. However, taking the boards can be stressful in itself, so I wanted to give you some tips so you will ace it on the first try. First and foremost, I highly recommend purchasing a study course to help prepare you for your upcoming board certification exam. There are a variety of study courses available for you to choose from. Courses may include content taught during an in-person class, or you may have access to an online program. Your study course will typically come with study materials and perhaps a guide book with practice test questions. Depending on how you learn, this may help guide you to the study course most suitable to you.

As far as study resources go, I've seen several websites that offer free study material or practice test questions. There are also plenty of board certification exam study books available for purchase, and I found a number of them on Amazon. You may also want to purchase material from different companies to have more variety while you study. When I was searching for study material I purchased a study course as well as several additional study books from different companies. Below I've listed a few resources to choose from when trying to find the best fit study course for you. This list is by no means all-inclusive so continue to do your research into what program or resources you prefer to use.

- Fitzgerald NP Certification Exam www.fhea.com. Dr. Margaret Fitzgerald is a seasoned nurse practitioner who offers a variety of courses through her website. Fitzgerald offers not only certificate exam study courses but an array of other resources as well.
- Barkley & Associates Curriculum Review www.npcourses.com. A comprehensive website that offers certification study courses in many different NP specialties.
- Advanced Practice Education Associates www.apea.com. This website offers anything from live classes to online courses and everything in between.
- Necessary Workshops www.necessaryworkshops.com. Offers both RN and NP preparation for certification as well as other helpful resources.
- Board Vitals www.boardvitals.com. Offers board certification prep courses as well as CE courses.

Renewal of Your Board Certification

You won't have to worry about this right away as you will have several years between taking your original board examination and renewing your board certification. However, I wanted to mention it so that you have it in the back of your mind and not have this come as a shock down the line.

Every few years (usually five years) you will have to renew your board certification. In order to do this, you will need to meet certain requirements. This may include but is not limited to: providing verification of clinical hours worked, completing a minimum amount of continuing education units (typically additional pharmacology continuing education units will be required), holding an active RN and NP license, and paying the applicable fee. If these requirements cannot be met, you may have to retake the examination. You definitely do not want to put yourself through taking the exam again so I suggest you keep on top of the requirements.

Nurse Practitioner License

Once you have graduated from your nurse practitioner program and have successfully passed your board certification for your specialty, you will be eligible for licensure to practice as a nurse practitioner in your state. Licensing is different from board certification in that it is on a state-by-state basis and is regulatory in nature. You are not allowed to practice in your state unless you hold an active license, both as an RN and as an NP.

Each state has different steps that need to be taken in order to apply for your nurse practitioner license once you graduate, so it is best to visit your state's board of nursing website for the most up-to-date and accurate information. For example, in certain states you will receive your prescriptive authority once you apply for your NP license, while in others you have to apply for it separately. In some states you can apply for RN and NP at the same time, while in other states you have to wait for your RN first before applying for your NP license. These little nuances can be confusing and I suggest you review the requirements in detail prior to applying in order to ensure you have all the necessary paperwork. I actually printed off the NP licensure requirements when applying and checked off everything I needed once I had completed it. This helped me to understand the process a bit better and I was able to be more organized.

Additionally, there is a great website where you can find information on your state's licensure requirements, which is www.nursinglicensure.org. I didn't discover this site until after I was already a licensed NP, but I wish I had as it would have made the process much smoother. There's a ton of information on this site from licensure requirements to collaborative relationships and everything in between. To clarify any confusion about your state NP license requirements you can also call or email your state board of nursing. In my experience, I've found them to be very helpful and they usually respond pretty quickly to inquiries.

Licensure in Other States

After you graduate you will most likely get your original NP license in the state where your school is located. However, you may then decide to move to another state; thus you will need to get licensed in whichever state that you move to. As I said earlier, some states allow you to apply for your RN and NP license at the same time. However, for those that don't you will need to apply for your RN first and then your NP license once you've obtained your RN license. Many but not all states participate in Nursys (www.nursys.com), which is an online verification tool that allows you to send verification of your nursing license to another state. It also lets employers and the public verify that you are a licensed nurse in a particular state.

The process of applying for an RN license and an NP license differs by state. For nurses located in certain states you are able to participate in the Enhanced Nurse Licensure Compact (eNLC), which recently transitioned from the original Nurse Licensure Compact (NLC). This means that if you hold an RN in a state that participates in the eNLC, you will be able to work as an RN in another state that is part of the eNLC without obtaining an additional state license, though you will be granted a multistate license by your home state. For more information on multistate RN licensure visit www.ncsbn.org/enlc. Although you cannot get a multistate license at this time as an NP, this is currently in process. At the time of this publication there were three states that had enacted APRN compact legislation; however, the compact will not go into effect until ten states have passed this legislation. For more information, you can visit www.aprncompact.com.

If you know that you will be moving to another state as soon as you complete your NP program, make sure to apply for your RN license well in advance. Depending on the state, your RN license may come relatively quickly or may take months. This is important to know because it will hold you up from working as an NP. Many of my colleagues applied for their RN license in the state where they were moving while we were still in our NP program. Thus, as soon as they passed their boards they were able to apply for their NP license without having to wait for their RN license first. Genius!

Miscellaneous

Below are a few more items that you may be applying for prior to starting your first nurse practitioner job.

Apply for Your DEA Number

You will need to obtain your Drug Enforcement Administration number also known as your DEA number. Although this application can be completed relative quickly, it may take weeks for you to get your actual DEA number in the mail, so I suggest not putting this off. A DEA number is not required to practice in your state; however, it is required if you are going to write prescriptions for controlled substances. Many employers will require you to hold an active DEA in that state in order to work for their organization. Having a DEA number is also a testament to how far NPs have come as we are able to write controlled substance prescriptions in all 50 states and in Washington, D.C. However, the state will determine which substances you can and cannot prescribe and may also limit the quantity you are allowed to prescribe.

Your employer may pay your DEA fee as part of your contract (more on this in the next chapter). However, if you pick up part-time or per diem work you usually have to pay out of pocket for it. At the time of this publication a DEA number fee for nurse practitioners was $731 for three years. This will most likely be one of your costlier NP expenses as state RN and NP licenses cost far less. For more information on obtaining a DEA number you can visit https://apps.deadiversion.usdoj.gov/webforms/

Apply for Your NPI (National Provider Identifier)

An NPI number is a number unique to a healthcare provider in the US that is issued by the Centers for Medicare and Medicaid Services. This is something you'll need to get prior to starting your first job. You can apply online for one at https://nppes.cms.hhs.gov/NPPES/Welcome.do

Malpractice Insurance

Most employers will provide you with some sort of malpractice insurance. This expense is optional if you are insured through your organization; however, many NPs opt to purchase their own personal malpractice insurance for peace of mind. I've heard lectures and read books by lawyers who suggest having your own malpractice insurance. I listened to their advice and have always kept my own malpractice insurance despite being insured by my employer. Even though it's an additional expense, it's definitely worth it. Many different companies offer plans that vary in cost depending on your specialty and other variables.

Keep Your Documents Organized

Now that we've discussed your obligations prior to starting your NP practice, let's look at how to keep them all organized. Before I graduated, my program director required all of us to scan specific paperwork onto a jump drive and we had to turn it in for verification. At the time, I thought that this was such as hassle as there were a lot of documents to keep track of and I didn't have a lot of spare time to do it. However, I found that scanning everything onto a jump drive and then into a folder on my computer has been incredibly helpful. By doing this I have been able to keep all of my important documents organized and in a location where they are easily accessible. I can't tell you how many times I've been asked to send in a professional document such as my state license or DEA number, and I was so glad it was all on a file on my computer where I could easily find it. I also suggest doing the same thing with all of your professional documents and recommend scanning the following items onto your computer as soon as you receive them.

- Preceptor evaluations. This is a great way to show your first potential employer how you performed in the clinical setting. Although you may never get asked to submit these evaluations, it's nice to have these forms available just in case.
- Letters of recommendation. I've kept almost every letter of recommendation ever written for me. I suggest you keep them handy as well, as you never know when you'll need one.
- Final transcript(s). All final transcripts, regardless of where you received them, should be scanned to your computer for easy access.
- Diploma(s).
- Licenses. This includes your RN and NP licenses as well as any other professional license that you may hold.
- Certifications. This may include but is not limited to ACLS, BLS, PALS, etc.
- Board certification. This is one of the many documents that you will have to submit to your employer prior to being hired. It's definitely one to keep on hand.
- DEA number. You will need to have this number handy. I also suggest writing it down in a safe place as you may need to provide it every now and again especially when writing controlled prescriptions.
- Awards, publications, and publicity you may have received.

- Continuing education certificates.
- Any other documents that you may have that pertain to your NP career.

The best way to do this is to scan everything into a file on your computer and label it accordingly. This will also be very useful if you move to another state and have several different state licenses to keep track of. I also recommend putting everything into a spreadsheet with license and certification expiration dates. This is important because if something expires before you have renewed it, this could really affect your job. I can't say it enough. Stay organized!

Join a Nurse Practitioner Organization

As a nurse practitioner, it's nice to stay connected with your peers by becoming a member of your state and/or national nurse practitioner organization. There are various professional nurse practitioner organizations available for you to join. From local chapters of large national organizations to specialty specific organizations, there's an NP organization out there for just about anybody. With all of these options available, you may even decide to become a member of multiple organizations.

At the state level, you may see that your state has multiple NP organizations, some that are regionally grouped. This is a great way to get to know like-minded professionals in your geographic area. They may have conferences or events that you can attend, and you are also able to network with other NPs. If your state has an NP organization (which it most likely does) I highly suggest you check it out. Not only will you meet other NPs who may turn into your friends, you may also be able to participate in some great events. At the national level, there are also various nurse practitioner organizations that you can join. These organizations tend to be much larger than the organizations at the state level; however, they still provide an abundance of resources for their members. Many NP organizations offer perks to members such as free CE courses, access to online and print journals, and discounts on conferences. They may also be actively involved in lobbying for nurse practitioner laws. Many of these organizations also have job boards and are a good resource to help with your job search.

Bonding with other nurse practitioners over your work, frustrations, accomplishments, and the challenges of medicine is priceless. Sometimes no one else besides another NP can really understand what you go through daily.

You may even meet lifelong friends through your professional membership. There is a list of both state and national NP organizations in the appendix. Although this list is comprehensive, it is not all-inclusive. I suggest doing additional research if you are interested in becoming a member of a professional NP organization.

Continuing Education

You will have to maintain continuing education (CE) credits to retain your nurse practitioner license and/or board certification. As a job perk, many employers will pay for your CE courses and give you paid days off to complete them. If you just graduated you won't need to worry about this right away; however, keep it in the back of your head as you don't want to get stuck having to scramble to complete your required CEs at the last minute. Obtaining CEs can be done in a variety of ways and below are a few of the ways in which continuing education units can be earned.

Attend a Continuing Education Conference

There are hundreds of conferences year-round all over the world that offer a wide variety of continuing education topics. Many times, they're held in beautiful locations and at nice hotels and resorts. They even have CE conferences on cruise ships! I haven't personally participated in a cruise CE; however, I've checked out their itineraries and they look pretty amazing. Just a quick online search will show you just how many CE conferences are available to you. As I mentioned above, your state and national NP organization will most likely offer CE conferences. As an NP, you don't just have to attend NP conferences; you can also attend conferences sponsored by other healthcare professionals such as physicians.

Online CEs

Many websites offer online CEs with some even offering free content! These are incredibly convenient as you can study from your own home when you have free time available. I did many of my CEs online as a member through my national NP organization. These were free with my membership, convenient, and I could learn from anywhere.

Precept Students

Being a preceptor is also another way to obtain continuing education units. As a preceptor, you will have the opportunity to have NP students shadow you, just as you shadowed your clinical preceptors when you were a student. Working as a preceptor is a great way to give back and educate students new to the profession. From what I have seen there can be a shortage of preceptors, and becoming a preceptor is a wonderful contribution to the profession. Some schools will even give tuition credit if you precept their students, which is a great way to pay for your education. I have never been a preceptor; however, one of my NP friends is a preceptor to both NP and medical students and really enjoys it.

As you've learned in this chapter there is a lot to think about between graduating from your nurse practitioner program and actually starting your first nurse practitioner job. This can be an incredibly exciting time but also filled with anxiety about what must be completed in order to practice as an NP. Everything you need to accomplish prior to starting your new career may seem overwheming. If there is any confusion about what you need to do before you start working you can always contact your state board of nursing, which is an excellent resource. You can also clarify questions with your school, which should be a good resource for information on state licensure requirements. When in doubt, ask! You don't want your license or other important documents to be held up due to a preventable mistake on your part.

· 7 ·

THE JOB HUNT

An organization, no matter how well designed, is only as good as the people who live and work in it.

—Dee Hock

This chapter is designed to help you find a job that is the "right fit" for you as well as guide you in negotiating the terms under which you are going to work. Once you have successfully completed your program and are nationally board certified and licensed to practice in your state, the world is your oyster and you will have many job opportunities available to you. If you are anything like me and didn't have a "real career" prior to becoming a nurse practitioner, you will find that this shift from struggling to find a job to being in high demand is a real game changer. There is no shortage of NP jobs available, and it only takes a brief scan of internet job postings to realize just how many jobs are out there.

When I say that the job you decide to take needs to be the "right fit" I don't say that lightly. As a nurse practitioner working in your profession, you may be offered several positions before deciding on which one to accept. I highly advise you to be very selective in this process. Remember, you will be spending a good portion of your time at your job and among your colleagues, and you want to enjoy your time there. I personally believe that it is important that you like what you do and with whom you work as this will greatly affect your job satisfaction. Of course, everyone has their bad days, and this is to be expected, but going to work each day dreading what is going to walk through the door or having anxiety about all the work that needs to be done is not a good feeling. Hence, choosing the right fit job from the beginning is crucial. Trust me because I've been there personally, and have had some NP jobs that were less than stellar. I suggest you choose wisely!

Never forget that as a nurse practitioner you will be in very high demand. You have also just spent the last several years getting to where you are and you deserve to love your job. If at all possible, try not to accept the first job offer unless you know it's the perfect job for you. This will give you time to feel out what else is available, and there may be an even better offer around the corner. I wish you the best of luck with your job search and hope you find an incredible position where you will grow both personally and professionally.

Job Search Resources

This next section is designed to help you with your nurse practitioner job search. This can be a very exciting time for you as you've just completed a rigorous program and are ready to yet again embark upon a new adventure. Nevertheless, you may be feeling anxiety about finding a job and beginning your practice as a new graduate.

Below I've created a list of several resources that will help you with your job search. This list, however, is not all-inclusive and I suggest you continue using all available resources to help you find a great position. Remember that there are thousands of options and resources available to help you with your search; you just need to find them! Don't forget to also checkout the comprehensive list of job resources in the appendix. You can refer back to chapter one, which also had quite a bit of information on NP jobs. Now, let's go find you a job!

Online Job Listings

If you simply type the phrase "nurse practitioner jobs" into any online search engine you will find thousands and thousands of positions available posted on multiple websites. You'll also notice once you've begun your search that there will be new jobs posted daily. There are so many nurse practitioner jobs available online that it's almost to the point of overwhelming!

Throughout my job search I used the internet as the primary source to look for job openings. Most sites I used were very user-friendly and had a great deal of information pertaining to the position. Since there are so many jobs, it might be a good idea to start off with a narrower criterion and then broaden your search. For example, you may type "family nurse practitioner jobs" instead of just "nurse practitioner jobs" into the search engine. That will narrow your search to NP jobs specifically for family NPs. Although this may remove jobs that you may be eligible to apply for, it will also eliminate other NPs jobs that do not pertain to you, thus making your search much easier. You may also be able to filter your search by part-time versus full-time or by salary requirements.

While I was starting my job search as newly graduated NP I used a variety of websites to help me. However, I found www.indeed.com and their smartphone app by far one of the most valuable resources in my job search. If you upload your resume, you can literally apply for jobs from anywhere using their smartphone app. Out to dinner with friends and see a job you love? Just a click of a button and your resume is sent to the employer just like that. So fast and so convenient!

Although I didn't necessarily get my job through this site, it taught me a lot about what types of jobs were available. Searching online also allows you to see what employers are offering in terms of salary and benefits. You can use this information to your advantage when negotiating for the position that you want. In the appendix, I've listed many websites that will help you with your online job search. Many of these sites also offer free smartphone apps, which I found very helpful because they allow you to apply for positions from anywhere.

Residency Programs

Although somewhat new to the profession, nurse practitioner residency programs have become increasingly popular as an option for new graduate nurse practitioners to pursue additional training prior to starting their first job. These residencies are usually paid, though the pay may be lower than an average NP salary.

Typically, as a resident, you are in a setting with mini-rotations to get more exposure to a wider variety of patients. The residency may be part of a major hospital or may be run by a local community health center. While you are not a student while in residency, you will most likely still have a preceptor or someone to consult with during the day while you see patients. Over the years a number of nurse practitioner residency programs have popped up, and even while writing this book I have heard of several more in the works. They are extremely competitive, so I suggest taking similar steps when applying to them as you did when you applied to your NP program.

Nurse practitioner residencies help transition the new graduate into clinical practice and are a great way to boost your clinical knowledge while getting hands-on work experience. If you are a recent graduate and are not ready to jump into a job without additional training, an NP residency may be a great fit for you. Below is a website that lists many of these residencies (and fellowship programs) currently available. This list may not be all-inclusive, so if a residency is what you're looking for I suggest doing additional research: www.bestmasterofscienceinnursing.com/great-nurse-practitioner-residen cy-programs.

Recruiters

Recruiters can be an excellent resource to help you find the job of your dreams. Essentially, it's their job to get you a job! However, the downside to recruiting agencies is that you can be bombarded with emails, calls, and even text messages if you post your resume online (this has happened to me on more than one occasion). I suggest if you want to work with a recruiter, pick an agency or two where you have found jobs that interest you. This way you may not be as inundated with people in search of your skills.

Some recruiters staff for permanent placement positions while others staff for locum tenens work. They may even find you a job that is temporary but could turn into a permanent position. I've communicated with a number of recruiters while searching for jobs and I've found that it comes down to work style. You'd like to find a recruiter who understands your needs and wants, and gets back to you on a timely schedule. Since you'll be working with this person to find a job and it may take time, it's important to have a good working relationship. I've actually chosen one agency over another because of the work ethic of one recruiter I met. He was very personable and helpful, and was often communicating with me regarding available jobs. For more information on NP recruitment companies I've included a list of agencies in the appendix for you to reference.

Locum Tenens

I briefly touched base on locum tenens in chapter one of this book. Locum tenens positions are designed to fill gaps in the system and typically look for temporary hires although there is a possibility your temporary job could turn into permanent placement. A locum tenens job could be as short as a few days or could be for months at a time, depending on the needs of the organization.

The organizations that recruit for locum tenens usually offer a variety of incentives for the job, which may include paid housing and travel accommodations. They also may pay for licensing and fees, and all of these perks add up, which can be incredibly lucrative. These jobs also offer you the opportunity to travel if you want, and typically help with the licensure process if you will need to get licensed in another state. If you do not want to feel bound to a long-term contract and want to try different organizations/health care settings before you settle on one, locum tenens may be a great option for you. Make sure to read the job description carefully as some of these positions do not hire new graduates.

A great travel NP blog that offers many tips is www.travelingnp.com. The blog was started by a locum tenens nurse practitioner who offers a ton of valuable information for those interested in pursuing this type of work. For more information on locum tenens agencies, check out the appendix for a list of resources.

HRSA Sites

If you have received a HRSA scholarship or are interested in loan repayment (previously discussed in chapter four), the HRSA website is the best place to begin your search. Visit their website for more information on available jobs and HRSA sites at https://connector.hrsa.gov.

It's important to note that not all available jobs are listed on this website, so if there is an organization where you'd like to work, you can also contact them directly. Additionally, numerical HPSA (Health Professional Shortage Areas) scores can change. These HPSA scores are designed to rank how underserved an area is with the highest score being the most underserved. If you have received a scholarship or loan repayment you may be required to work at a site with a certain HPSA score (or higher). I suggest that if there is a site where you are considering working, you should make sure and call the agency just to double check what site number they are. Sites may have different HPSA scores for primary care, dental, and mental health services.

Although the above-mentioned site is very useful to help locate a HRSA site, you can still find loan repayment sites on just about any online job board. While looking for a job that was a HRSA site I would type in "nurse practitioner loan repayment," which would bring up any NP jobs that offered loan repayment options. This was a quick way for me to filter out sites that did not qualify so that both the potential employer and I did not waste our time.

Word of Mouth

Now I hate to sound cliché by advising you to go out and network to find a job; however, I've learned from personal experience that it works. Putting the word out there that you're looking for work can really help you get a job, often very quickly. Not because it's about "who you know" but really because it's about "hearing about open positions and employers in need of NPs." Prior to graduating I kept hearing about different places that needed providers. Once I actually was licensed, I was constantly asked if I was available to work or if I knew any other nurse practitioners who would like to pick up extra work. I received my first two NP jobs by word of mouth. One was through a clinical position that turned into a per diem job, and the other was through a classmate of mine as the place where she was working needed additional providers. So why word of mouth? So a potential employer can find a great NP!

Additional Resources

As you have come to see in this chapter, nurse practitioners are in demand! There are literally thousands of jobs available to choose from daily. Now let's talk about a few other additional resources that weren't previously mentioned that may help you find a job.

- *University job fairs.* While you're a student you may have potential employers come to your academic institution to participate in a job fair. This is a great way to discuss their organization without any pressure to make a decision about employment. Think of it as a meet and greet where you can discuss potential work opportunities. Make sure to dress appropriately when attending these fairs. You may also want to bring copies of your CV to give to an organization that interests you.

- *Nursing/nurse practitioner journals and magazines.* You may find jobs advertised in these magazines so make sure to give them a once over if you have any on hand.
- *State and national nurse practitioner organizations.* As I've said previously, both state and national NP associations typically have a career section that will list NP jobs. I encourage you to check these out as your future job may be one of those listed!
- *Private organizations.* If there is an organization where you'd like to work you can usually find their list of jobs posted online. Check the job boards of companies, hospitals, or universities where you'd like to work. Chances are they have NP positions available. If they don't they may have positions opening up in the near future.

Job Search Challenges

Now that we've reviewed how to find a job, let's look at potential challenges you may face while applying for your first NP position. Despite the fact that there are thousands of nurse practitioner jobs available all over the planet, landing that initial job may still be a challenge. You may find yourself taking all the needed steps such as perfecting your CV and networking within your social circles, and still may have discovered that you are unable to secure that first position. I've know people who haven't been able to find work for whatever reason for a long time, and it can become very discouraging. This next section highlights some of the ways the job search may be challenging and what to do if you encounter obstacles. Try not to get too frustrated if this happens to you; remember that you will eventually get hired, but it may just take a little more time.

No New Graduates

One of the most frustrating aspects about starting your job search as a brand-new graduate is that you may not even be able to apply to a number of positions because you are a newly graduated NP. While spending quite a bit of time looking for jobs right after I had graduated, I came across a number of positions that I was ineligible to apply for because I was a new graduate. It seemed as if every other job description I encountered had the phrase "no new graduates." At the time, this was very frustrating to me; however, now that

I've been in the field for a while I realize that such statements by employers are a good thing. You don't want to work somewhere that doesn't support you as a new graduate as this can turn into a bad situation.

If you see this phrase or something along these lines in the job listings just continue on with your search. Even if the job seems perfect for you, don't worry, another perfect job will come around again. Although there are plenty of jobs that are not open to new graduates, the opposite is also true where you will see the phrase "open to new grads." This can definitely be used to your advantage, and some employers actually prefer new graduates as they are able to train you themselves.

Lack of Experience

Another phrase you may come across frequently during your job search is "needs to have X amount of experience." This could be a certain number of years of experience that an employer wants you to have for the position. Or perhaps they would like you to have experience in a particular area of medicine such as the emergency room. Again, this can be challenging because as a new graduate you won't have any NP experience.

Nevertheless, there are ways you may be able to compensate for this, and you can still market yourself accordingly. If you worked as an RN in a particular setting, you could highlight this experience you had. I find that this is most often true for RNs with acute care experience who end up going on to work in the emergency department (ED) or ICU as NPs. Or perhaps you did volunteer work in a certain setting, and you may be able to emphasize those transferable skills you learned.

Location

Sometimes the challenge of finding a job comes down to your physical location. If you live in a rural community, finding a job may be harder than in a large urban city. Or on the other hand, perhaps you are living in an urban area in an already saturated market with a lot of competition, and there aren't many available jobs left. If you cannot relocate for a position you may have to make compromises such as commuting in order to accept the position. Or you may need to accept a position in a specialty that you wouldn't have chosen otherwise. If you are having trouble getting work due to your area of residence, there are other options available, which may include telemedicine, online teaching, and locum tenens NP positions. Remember, there's always a solution, but sometimes you just have to get creative to find it.

———————

If you find yourself unable to get a job right out of school I suggest you take a step back and look at what might be hindering you. Perhaps your CV needs to be cleaned up, or you need to reevaluate your references. Maybe you need to work on your interviewing skills. Whatever the challenge is, by pausing and reevaluating the situation, you may soon discover what is blocking you from that first new position. Additionally, it wouldn't hurt to reach out to a recruiter to help you with your first placement. Their job is to get you hired, and working with a recruiter may be the answer to your predicament.

Negotiating and Accepting a Job Offer

Congratulations on being offered a job (or multiple jobs) as a nurse practitioner! After determining that the position is a good fit for you, the next step is contract negotiation and finally accepting that long-awaited offer. Make sure to read your contract (or offer letter) thoroughly and carefully. Clarify anything that you don't understand and if both parties agree on changes, get it in writing. If something is missing that you think should be included and it is negotiated into the offer, again get it in writing! You get the point—you need everything written down!

Some of the items below may not be applicable to you; however, these are the basic items that a standard contract or offer letter should include. If not in the contract, then some of the points below should be in the employee handbook for you to reference. Don't ever let someone pressure you into signing a contract that you don't feel comfortable signing. You don't want to sign something that down the line you wish you hadn't, or not receive something you thought you were going to. And again, read everything carefully! While negotiating a contract make sure your employer includes the following information:

- Compensation. Will you be paid hourly or salary? Will you be paid extra if you agree to work more? Will you get paid more if you see more patients? Will you get a bonus after working there for a certain amount of time? What days of the month will you be paid? Understand clearly what your compensation is and how it's structured. Make sure this is all openly articulated in your contract or offer letter. This will help to prevent any misunderstandings down the line.

- Continuing education allowance. Many employers pay for continuing education as part of your contract. However, this is not standard practice for locum tenens employees and is usually reserved for permanent placement opportunities. You may be allotted a certain amount of money and time away from direct patient care to complete this. Many employers will pay for the education itself plus travel expenses and lodging.
- Licensing and fees. Will your potential employer pay for your RN and NP license fees? Will they pay for your license renewal? Will they pay for your DEA fee? CPR recertification? All these fees add up and are not cheap. It's good to know beforehand if your employer will pay for or reimburse you for your professional fees, and if so, which ones.
- Benefits. These may include health insurance, dental insurance, life insurance, and 401k plan. Other questions to ask include will your spouse and family be covered under your insurance plan? If so, will their plan need to be paid for out of your pocket? Will your employer match your contributions for your retirement plan? When will your benefits start? If not on day one, how long must you be an employee to start receiving them? Some other benefits may be discounts on gym membership, your cell phone bill, and other perks your company may offer.
- Paid time off (PTO). Do you get vacation days? Sick days? Paid holidays? Personal days? If so, how many per year? If you don't use it all, will PTO roll over to the next year? If so, how many days will be allotted to carryover? What about maternity leave? If your paid time off is not ideal, can you negotiate for more time off?
- Schedule. Will you work days? Nights? Four 10-hour days? Five 8-hour days? Three 12-hour days? Full-time? Part-time? Weekends? Many job sites will post positions with the hours they would like you to work. However, from my experience this is definitely a negotiable area that you can tweak. If you find a job that you love but the schedule doesn't fit, feel free to talk to your potential employer about changing it. This may not always be possible, for example if the job is for nights and you prefer to work days. However, it is worth having a discussion as you may be able to come to an agreement that works for both you and your employer.

- Location. Will you be located at just one site, or will be you be required to travel to multiple sites? If you are required to travel, will they cover your mileage?
- Administrative (admin) Time. This is designated time that you may be allotted each week to finish administrative tasks and does not involve patient care. I've never had this as an option, but one of my NP friends has. The longer she works at the organization, the more admin time she can negotiate for. It's definitely a much-desired perk!
- Patients per day. This is an incredibly important question to ask as the number of patients you see will impact your practice. Are you required to see a certain number of patient's daily? If you don't see the required number of patients per day are you penalized? Will you get paid for additional patient visits above your requirement? Will your daily average be eight patients a day or are you expected to see twenty-five patients a day? Clarify this.
- Malpractice insurance. This is included in most standard offers for both permanent placement and locum tenens positions. However, as I've mentioned previously, regardless whether your employer pays your malpractice, it's still a good idea to have your own.
- On-call. Will your position require you to be on-call? And if so, how often? Will you be expected to go into the facility if you are on call to see the patient, or is it triage only?
- Dress code. Are you required to wear scrubs? Business casual? If you wear a white coat or scrubs, does your facility get your uniform laundered? If you have tattoos are they allowed to be visible?
- Moving allowance. If you are moving for the job be sure to inquire about a moving allowance. Some employers provide this, while others do not. Some will pay for moving expenses if you agree to work a certain amount of time, and if you leave before this time period, you may have to pay it back.
- Non-compete clauses. This may be included as part of your contract and is designed to prevent you from working for competitors. For example, your contract may state that you are not allowed to work for one year within a 25-mile radius of your current site. From what I've learned about non-compete clauses it is best to avoid signing this type of contract. If your employer will not remove this clause, I suggest trying to negotiate for less radius/time. If the above example is in your

contract perhaps you can negotiate the clause to state for six months, or within a ten-mile radius.

- Resignation. How much notice are you required to give prior to your resignation. Will you be involved in training your replacement? Will they pay you back your PTO days that you haven't used?

Other Considerations

Aside from negotiating a contract there are other things to consider at your potential place of employment. Remember to consider each point carefully. You will be spending a large part of your time at work, and your happiness and job satisfaction are important.

- Facility setting. Will you be working inpatient or outpatient? Is the setting private practice? Community Health Clinic? Rural? Urban? I could go on and on about facility settings, but you get the point that there are many types of facilities out there. Depending on your training and experience you may prefer one setting over another. This is important to consider when accepting a job offer.
- Patient population. What kind of patients will you be seeing? Underserved? Geriatrics? If you will be in a family practice setting, how many patients will be chronic care? Pediatrics? You may already know what kind of patient population you want to work with. However, if not, you may learn this quickly on the job. If you already know there is a certain patient population you don't want to work with, I highly suggest not taking that position.
- Type of care provided. Will you be expected to perform procedures? If so, which ones? Chronic care? Acute sick visits? A little of both? If you will be entering a setting where you will be required to provide care or perform procedures that you are not familiar with, clarify that someone there will help train you.
- Staffing. Will there be other medical providers onsite? If so, how many? Physicians? NPs? PAs? Is there another provider at your facility who could mentor you if needed? Will you be working all alone in a clinic? I don't recommend this for newly graduated NPs as you will want all the available support you can get when starting your practice. Will you have a nurse or medical assistant working with you? If so, how many support staff are available?

- Morale and work culture. Do the staff like their jobs? Do you hear people complaining if you go visit the site? Do staff spend time together outside of work? Do employees seem happy? Although you cannot judge what your experience will be like by comparing it with others, you can evaluate if any red flags indicate future problems.
- Respect of the nurse practitioner profession. This may seem like a no-brainer but I recommend you evaluate how your potential employer and colleagues feel about NPs. Do you get the sense that they will treat you as a colleague? Or will you be treated as a "physician extender" where you won't be able to autonomously manage your patients? Not that you should necessarily care about their opinions, but understanding this will guide how you will practice and how much autonomy you will have within the organization.

Additional Nurse Practitioner Positions

Aside from working as a nurse practitioner in a clinical facility, there are many other roles that nurse practitioners hold. I don't necessarily recommend taking on a position aside from a clinical one right after graduation as you will need hands-on experience. A friend of mine, however, did take on an administrative role without patient care right after he graduated and is doing quite well. Nonetheless, the majority of recent NP graduates will be pursing clinical work upon graduation, but keep in mind that the list below provides options that may be a good fit in the future.

Nurse Practitioner Faculty

As the nursing and nurse practitioner profession continues to expand, the need for both RN and NP faculty has increased exponentially. There is a large market for nursing faculty to teach nursing and nurse practitioner students. If you like teaching and want to positively influence the next generation of nurses or nurse practitioners you may enjoy working in a faculty position. The educational role could include being an academic professor, clinical preceptor, director of a nurse practitioner program, and mentoring students. There is even a loan repayment option available for nursing faculty, which was discussed in chapter four.

As many schools are opting to provide online programs, many of these faculty positions are done remotely. Basically, this means that if hired as a professor, you may be able to work from virtually anywhere in the world! This offers a lot of flexibility for those who cannot move for a position or who may have a family schedule they need to work around. Working as nurse or nurse practitioner faculty for a university offers a wide variety of options and I suggest you evaluate each job description carefully to make sure you like the role.

Administrative Positions

While this can also overlap with a university faculty position, many NPs also work in administrative roles that may or may not hold a clinical component. Several of my NP friends have worked at a clinic where the medical director was an NP. This may be an option for you once you've had extensive clinical experience, but it's definitely not for the new graduate. However, I wanted to mention this so you get an idea of some of the other types of positions available.

NPs who work in administrative roles may be involved with tasks such as business development of the organization, improving clinical workflow, or working on quality improvement of an organization. Nurse practitioners can also be found managing and supervising other NPs as well as other staff. If you decide to take on an administrative role you will find a wide range of options.

Telemedicine

Telemedicine, also known as telehealth, allows healthcare professionals to provide medical services virtually to patients. This is typically done with face-to-face video conferencing or a telephone call. As healthcare organizations continue to expand their services, telemedicine has become an increasingly popular way to reach more patients, especially those who have trouble leaving their home to come to the clinic. Telemedicine has become widespread and there are often positions available to nurse practitioners to see patients remotely. Once you feel comfortable with your diagnosis and management skills, working in telemedicine can be a great way to supplement your income or just to be able to work from home. I've also seen nurse practitioners start their own telemedicine practices, which is also an option for you down the line if you want to be your own boss. The sky's the limit with telemedicine because with an increase in globalization, even the most rural patients are able to connect with a healthcare provider.

Self-Employment

While this may not be the best option right away as you still need to build up your clinical skills, owning your own business may be your dream. More and more I see nurse practitioners opening their own clinical practices, especially as state practice barriers have been eliminated. Seeing NP-owned clinical practices makes me incredibly proud of the profession and shows just how far we've come in a little over half a century. If this is the route you will eventually be taking, I suggest that you contact your state board of nursing to see if there are certain requirements you must meet. Will you need a physician collaborator? Will someone need to review your charts? What are the legal requirements you must complete prior to opening up your practice?

Aside from the board of nursing, additional considerations include creating the right entity to run your business such as an LLC (limited liability company) or other entity, creating a budget, purchasing the correct malpractice insurance, hiring staff, renting a location for your practice, marketing, logo, etc. You'll also need to hire a lawyer and an accountant. Going into business for yourself can be a dream career for many and if this is your goal more power to you. I also suggest finding a mentor or someone who has already done it so you don't have to reinvent the wheel. Yes, you'll make mistakes, but a mentor will help guide you to prevent many of them.

Politics

To get from where we started as a profession over half a century ago to where we are today involved not only clinical care but political work as well. There are many NPs who lobby for changing outdated laws and try to make changes on both a state and national level to better serve the entire profession. There are also NPs who work for NP organizations that advocate for political change. If you'd like to get involved politically I suggest checking out the extensive list of NP organizations in the appendix.

——————

Throughout this chapter we've looked at how to transition from being a student nurse practitioner to a full-fledged practicing nurse practitioner clinician. As you can see from the previous pages there is a lot to consider prior to accepting your first NP job. If you're feeling overwhelmed by all the things you need to do, I suggest that you take a step back and take a deep breath. Reread this chapter to see if anything else can help you along the way, as there may be something you missed the first time. Once you've started your NP practice, you've embarked upon a whole other journey as a nurse practitioner. Now that you know a bit more about how to get a job and what types of positions are available, let's now look at what it will be like for you once you begin your practice.

· 8 ·

BRINGING IT ALL TOGETHER

Go forth and set the world on fire.

—St. Ignatius of Loyola

If you've made it to this part in the book and you've already finished your program, taken your board certification examination, and accepted your first NP position then you deserve a HUGE congratulations! You've accomplished an incredible amount and I encourage you to pause and reflect on how far you've come on your path. Sometimes we can get so focused on the end result that we forget about all the blood, sweat, and tears it took to get there. All the hard work and sacrifice that you've put in over the last few years have culminated in a lifelong career, one you will hopefully love and that will provide you with much personal satisfaction.

Although you've accomplished an incredible amount to get to this point, the journey as a practicing nurse practitioner has just begun. There are so many things that you have yet to learn and this can seem overwhelming at times. This chapter is not meant to provoke fear or anxiety about starting your practice, but rather to prepare you for what you don't learn in school. I've also shared some of my own tips for how to cope with stressors that are a part of the job. Remember, life will also hand us stress and there will always be bumps in the road; your job is to know yourself and use the tools available to best manage these situations once they arise. As the Greek philosopher Epictetus said, "It's not what happens to you, but how you react to it that matters."

My first NP job was working as a per diem NP at a women's health clinic in midtown Manhattan. Prior to my first day on the job, I had three days of training with the physician who owned the practice. We trained at her other private practice so I wasn't even familiar with the office until I arrived for my first shift. That quick training included everything from learning how to use the electronic medical record to practice protocols, billing, and of course how to diagnose and manage the patients.

That first day of work as a nurse practitioner was terrifying. It was such a whirlwind; I saw seventeen patients in about a five-hour time span. This is a lot of patients to see even for an experienced provider! Not only was I overwhelmed with the patient load, but to make matters more challenging I was the sole provider there. The physician/owner of the practice was not there for me to ask questions. Yes, I could contact her via the phone or by text, but it wasn't the same as having someone physically there to consult with. Suddenly it was time to sink or swim, and I chose to swim.

Preferably this is not the way that you want to start your career; however, looking back I learned an incredible amount, and I'm proud of how I managed under such duress. Not only was I able to diagnoses and treat the patients, but I also learned how to direct staff as well as step into a role of leadership. Friends of mine shared similar experiences during their first days, weeks, and months in their new role as nurse practitioner. All of a sudden there is this drastic transition from student to provider, and all the responsibilities that go with it can be quite overwhelming.

A common phrase I've heard repeated is "I have no idea what I'm doing." This may be true to a certain extent; however, many times you know more than you think you do. Remember, you're not the first nurse practitioner (or any other healthcare provider for that matter) to feel inept in managing patients, and you certainly won't be the last. Ideally you won't be starting off your nurse practitioner career in the same way that I did, but if you do, take a deep breath and as the popular phrase reminds us, "Keep calm and carry on."

On the other side of the spectrum, even seasoned NPs who change jobs to work with a completely different patient population or in an entirely new clinical setting can find themselves facing similar feelings. I recently spoke with an inpatient NP regarding a mutual patient. She stated she'd been an outpatient NP for many years and had recently switched jobs to work inpatient. She mentioned the challenges she faced, and starting her new position was a "whole new ball game," something completely different from her previous experiences. If you find yourself changing clinical settings, remember that there will always be a period of adjustment. Getting out of our comfort zones is scary, but it's what ultimately creates growth. Wherever you are in your nurse practitioner career give yourself the compassion and patience that you would give a close friend during these times of transition.

Beginning Your Practice

Promise me you'll always remember: you're braver than you believe, and stronger than you seem, and smarter than you think.

—A. A. Milne

As indicated above, starting off as a new graduate nurse practitioner can be a very scary feeling. After being in school and under the guidance of your professors and preceptors, you are finally able to spread your wings and fly. No more preceptors to consult with on patients or professors with whom you can review challenging cases. This feeling is incredibly rewarding as you've come so far on your journey but it is also very intimidating. Having the ability to take care of patients is a privilege and we must do right by them.

A new graduate definitely lacks a lot of knowledge and clinical skills so it can be nerve-wracking to think that other people's healthcare is in your hands. An NP I met a few years ago told me that by choosing to become a nurse practitioner, you are choosing to self-educate. We don't have as extensive schooling or training as physicians do. We also don't have mandatory residencies, which I think would greatly benefit the profession. This phrase about self-education has stuck with me throughout the years. It keeps me motivated to pursue educating myself for both the benefit of my patients and myself professionally.

Unfortunately, although you are a newly graduated NP, you may still be expected to hit the ground running. Many hiring managers don't realize that, unlike physicians, we don't have as extensive training, or the above-mentioned residencies. This means that as a new graduate you are expected to jump right in and expected to know how to manage the patients, some of whom have complex medical conditions. This can lead to feeling very intimidated, which is why I earlier emphasized the importance of choosing your first job very wisely. You want to make sure that your future employer knows your skillsets and is willing to work with you on the advancement of your skills. If you emphasize to your employer that you need time to adjust or a bit more training, they may be more flexible with your training schedule as you learn how to manage your patient load.

On the Job Tips

Now that you've actually started your job, there will be a whole new learning curve. Thus, I've created the following points, which are designed to help you successfully make this transition from nurse practitioner student to practicing clinician. These points are not all-inclusive so please feel free to add your own ways to become a successful NP.

Find a Mentor

Although this is definitely not required to start your career, I highly suggest finding a mentor, or if you're lucky finding more than one! From my own personal experience, having a mentor has been such a blessing and I'm so grateful to all of the wonderful healthcare providers who have mentored and taught me throughout the years. A mentor can be an experienced colleague at work whom you can ask for advice or a healthcare professional you can call to run questions by over the phone. During my time as an NP I've had multiple mentors, some of whom I've worked with in person and others who were only a phone call or text message away. The relationship you have with your mentor doesn't necessarily need to be a formal one either. It may just involve having that other medical provider available to ask the occasional clinical question. The more seasoned you are in your practice, the less you will be calling on your mentor. However, regardless of where you are in your practice, it's nice to have someone to look to for guidance.

Mentors don't necessarily have to be nurse practitioners; they can also come from other health disciplines such as physicians or PAs (I've had all three!). I encourage you to choose someone who is experienced in their practice as well as someone who shares your philosophy on healthcare. It wouldn't be in your benefit to have a mentor who doesn't know what they are doing, or who doesn't treat their patients in a kind and compassionate manner. A mentor should be someone with whom you feel safe discussing patient cases, as well as someone who won't act bothered or annoyed with your questions. The last thing you want is to have a mentor who doesn't want to be one, so choose your mentor wisely!

Having a compassionate and knowledgeable mentor in your place of employment is probably the most helpful type of mentorship available. I've been very fortunate to work with some amazing clinicians whom I can ask for help, advice, treatment plans, or a second opinion. Many times I've been incredibly grateful to have a colleague available to run a clinical question by or come in to see a patient with me when I had questions. Unfortunately, some of your colleagues may not want to take on this role to answer your questions and help you through tough clinical cases, and it's not their job either. They may find it a nuisance to help you as it may increase their workload. However, you'll find that some of your colleagues love to teach and really do enjoy mentoring someone new to the field.

If there is no one who can act as a mentor where you are working, you may want to check with your local NP organization. They may have nurse practitioners who will be more than happy to mentor you. Go ahead and give it a shot; you'll never know if you don't ask.

Use Your Resources

Once you're in clinical practice you'll need to be quick on your toes and make swift decisions regarding the medical management of your patients. From deciding what medication is best for your patient, to trying to figure out the best course of action for an incredibly complicated patient, you may need to use multiple resources to reach the answer. With the internet and smartphones at our fingertips, a lot of this information is only a few clicks away. The medical information on the internet is extensive, so you'll need to know which sites are legit and which you should avoid. Academic websites are key. To be honest with you I could not have survived without Uptodate! Aside from the internet there are many great books, journal articles, apps, and guidelines to help you manage your patients. Regardless of the information available, treating and managing patients is not just a science but an art as well. The answer you're looking for may not necessarily come from an external source but from the clinical intuition you will gain with experience.

For tough clinical questions, when I'm in a crunch I always know that I can ask someone for advice. Blessed are my co-workers and wonderful NP friends whom I can ask questions day or night. Even while they are managing their own patients, my NP friends are always willing to answer my questions. They may be too busy to answer me right away (but usually eventually do), and I've realized that friends and colleagues don't mind helping a fellow clinician out.

I often find myself texting or calling friends with clinical questions if they have more expertise in that clinical area than I do. For example, one of my friends is a fabulous acute care NP who works in a prominent NYC hospital. If I have questions about this area of medicine I'll ask for her advice as she has extensive expertise in that arena. Another friend is very knowledgeable about travel medicine, so any questions I have regarding this area of medicine, I ask her. You get it: ask the appropriate questions to the appropriate people!

Have Confidence—Know What You Know and Don't Know

Being able to treat patients confidently is not a skill that comes overnight, and it may take a while (even years) to feel comfortable with your clinical decision-making skills. As a newly graduated nurse practitioner you will find yourself questioning many decisions you make and often wondering if you treated the patient appropriately. You may find yourself thinking of them long after they have left your care. I've spent many nights wondering if there was something more I could have done for a particular patient or worrying about a sick patient's health.

Confidence also means knowing what you know and knowing what you don't know. I've personally witnessed arrogant healthcare providers providing patient care that they shouldn't have due to incorrectly thinking they knew how to appropriately manage that patient. Be confident but stay humble. If you don't know how to manage a patient don't pretend you do; it may put you into a situation you don't wish to be in and can set you up for a lawsuit. If I have a challenging patient that I don't know what to do with and can't find the answer, I will refer that patient to another provider. As the old saying goes, "It's better to be safe than to be sorry."

Working as an NP also means learning how to be decisive, a necessary skill that I mentioned earlier. This is something that I've struggled with personally but have gotten better at over time. As a new NP, I often took a long time to reach decisions that would best benefit my patient. I'd constantly question and analyze my decisions, not really feeling 100% sure of myself. Once I had been in practice for a while I gradually gained more confidence and realized I'd been making great decisions for my patients all along; it was just the confidence I lacked. The need for quick decision-making can put a lot of pressure on you, and you may doubt yourself. Your skills will come with experience, so be patient with yourself. For me, a big personal accomplishment was when I realized I didn't need to look up each patient case on Uptodate!

Openly Communicate with Your Employer

If you're feeling overwhelmed in your new NP position be sure to discuss your feelings with your employer. You don't want the little stressors to build up over time as this is not good for anyone involved. Depending on where you work, open communication with your boss may not be so easy. I've had employers who were not supportive of what I've needed, which is a horrible feeling. I've been put in positions where I felt incredibly uncomfortable, and the only way to fix the situation was to leave the practice, which I eventually did. On the other hand, I've had employers who were very supportive of me and who addressed all of my concerns. It can go either way, and if you find yourself working for someone you don't feel supported by, you may want to consider looking for another position.

Stand Up for Yourself

As a nurse practitioner, unfortunately many times you are not allotted the same respect as your physician colleagues. Even though you are working side by side providing the same services to the same patient population, because you are not a doctor you may hear the occasional negative comment from a colleague or patient. Regardless if it's a patient who won't see you because you're an NP, or a colleague who doesn't respect your role, it's imperative that you stand up for yourself (respectfully of course) and show those who doubt just what an awesome NP you are.

I recently had a new patient who started complaining that he had to see NPs at a sister clinic. After I informed him that I was also an NP, he became angry and got up to leave, proceeding to complain to me about the profession in general. He became aggressive and was escorted to the lobby where he continued his show. This incident made me really upset and while I was discussing it with my husband he wondered why I was taking it so personally. To him this guy was out of his mind and it didn't matter what he thought as his opinion was meaningless. He asked me, "Are you the voice of the NPs?" and I thought about it for a moment and said that heck yes I was! We all have to be the voice of the profession; it's what got us to where we are today.

Consider Specializing

Although I work in primary care and do not have a specialty at this point in my career, I have many NP friends who work in specialty fields and are really rocking it. Only one of them actually has subspecialty education in the field in which he works, while the rest learned their specialty on the job.

One of my good friends is an FNP but works in neurology, specifically movement disorders such as Parkinson's. She essentially works in a subspecialty of a specialty, which as you can imagine does not have as many healthcare providers as those working in family practice clinics. My friend could market herself to neurology clinics all over the country because having that sort of specialty knowledge is very valuable. She recently accepted an excellent position at a major hospital across the country, where she was referred to as a "unicorn," someone very rare in their field. Another FNP friend of mine has a HIV subspecialty degree and was just sought out by a major academic institution to work for them. He was offered an amazing position and benefits package for his specialty knowledge. These are just two of the many NPs who have chosen a specialty they enjoy and are really good at. I haven't found mine just yet, but I'll let you know when I do!

You may decide while in school what area of medicine you really love working in and go from there. Or you may work a few years before deciding that you would like to specialize in a certain area or with a certain patient population. If so, you may find yourself being scouted out for your specialty knowledge.

Surviving the Stress

Courage doesn't always roar, sometimes it's the quiet voice at the end of the day whispering I will try again tomorrow.

—Mary Anne Radmacher

I love the above quote because it's exactly how I feel some days after a long day of patient care when I'm just so drained that I want to fall into bed at 6:00 p.m. Many nurse practitioners, or any healthcare professional for that matter, may also be feeling similar emotions due to stress and fatigue. This can at times be overwhelming, especially to someone who is new to the field. From taking care of patients to dealing with staff, there are definitely some days when you will want to pull your hair out! Nevertheless, you can successfully manage all of the challenges thrown at you; it just takes some practice and learning how to use the tools and resources available to you. Below I've given a few tips on how to best manage on-the-job stress. Again, this list is not all-inclusive, and if there's anything that needs to be added for you to best manage your stress, put it on the list!

Managing Your Workload

It is my personal opinion that being able to manage your workload will set you up for great professional success. I'm an idealist and went into this profession because I wanted to take care of patients and to help people, especially underserved communities. However, there is so much more that comes with the job aside from face to face interactions in the exam room. Unfortunately, these tasks take up much more of your time than providing direct patient care. These responsibilities may include billing for services rendered, paperwork (lots and lots of paperwork), returning patient phone calls, referrals, reviewing lab results and imaging, prescription refills, signing documents, consulting other healthcare providers regarding mutual patients, meetings, and everyone's least favorite—the endless amounts of charting. It is unfortunate that more time is spent on these other obligations than with the patient; however, that is how the system is, and this is the world we live in today.

If you find the workload has become overwhelming, speak with your boss immediately to see if you can have administrative time, which as mentioned earlier, is time set aside allowing you to complete these tasks. Some organizations do not allow this, while others provide you with more admin time the longer you've been there. Depending on your employer you may be able to request additional time for patient office visits, negotiate for more autonomy to control your schedule, or anything else you think would help lighten your load. Remember, if you don't ask you won't know what can be done to help set you up to better manage your workload.

Avoiding Lawsuits

In today's litigious society, unfortunately, many nurse practitioners also practice with the threat of malpractice. Although the risk for NPs in general is low, it's still in the back of many practicing NPs minds. To alleviate this stress and as I've stated multiple times throughout the text, I highly advise that you purchase your own personal malpractice insurance. This not only legally helps protect you but also may bring some peace of mind. You may also want to research articles and books on ways to avoid malpractice as an NP. I've read some great literature on the subject and there are CEs on avoiding malpractice as well. You'll learn ways to protect yourself in the clinical arena, effectively setting you up for success.

Compassion Fatigue

Many NPs also suffer from compassion fatigue, that is, bearing witness to the traumas dealt with by their patients daily. Anyone who has sat with a patient crying over a new cancer diagnosis or comforted someone who cannot afford his prescription medications can attest to this. Some days can be overwhelming as each patient who comes to see you has a sadder story than the previous one. Their stories are incredibly heartbreaking and humbling, and just hearing what some of your patients go through can really tear you up inside. Sometimes there is nothing you can do besides offering an ear to listen while giving them your undivided attention. Sometimes it's enough, and sometimes it isn't.

For me, this kind of energy exchange is incredibly draining and I advise that you protect yourself from this type of emotional harm. This can mean taking a few minutes for yourself to regroup after a particularly challenging encounter or mentally visualizing yourself being shielded from any negativity permeating your energy field. You also need to realize that you can't solve everyone's problems, something that may be hard to accept. As an NP, you want to help your patients and fix whatever ailment they present with, but sometimes you just can't and realizing this can be freeing. Do whatever you need to do to keep yourself from being physically and mentally drained as a result of compassion fatigue.

Have Fun

Ok, you may be thinking, have fun? How can I have fun with all the challenges I may encounter? However, having fun on the job will help maintain the balance and minimize on-the-job stressors. If you love what you do and are in the right position, ideally it should be fun as well! Yes, there will be moments of stress and anxiety, but there will also be moments of fun, laughter, and joy. From laughing with your patient over a funny story he just told you, to spending time with your coworkers, you can find moments of joy and fun throughout the day.

I'm a jokester and love to have a good laugh with my patients, sometimes at my own expense. Recently a patient I'd only seen for the second time asked me if I'd given birth. Um, no, I had not given birth, and no, I wasn't pregnant the last time you saw me! She said she thought I had been and that now I looked really good. Thanks, I think. Anyway, we both had a good laugh over that one, and at least I was making progress in my physical appearance!

Taking Care of Yourself

When a person decides to become a nurse, they make the most important decision of their lives. They choose to dedicate themselves to the care of others.
—Margaret Harvey

You'll notice that the above quote speaks to nurses dedicating their lives to taking care of others, but nothing is said of nurses taking care of themselves. Although "take care of yourself" sounds like one of the oldest clichés out there, I can't express how true I think this sentiment is. As nurse practitioners, our job is to take care of patients, day in and day out. It doesn't matter what is going on with you in your personal life as your priority is the patient. In order to be there fully for a patient, you must "show up" and be present, regardless of what emotions or feelings you may have that day. This can be challenging at times as we all have things going on in our personal lives. But being present for your patients and really listening to them can make all the difference.

As Yoko Ono once said, "Healing yourself is connected with healing others." For us to be fully present and be there for our patients we must take care of ourselves first and foremost.

Self-Care

I liken self-care to the oxygen mask scenario on an airplane. If oxygen is low and the masks are dispensed, you're supposed to put yours on first before putting the mask on your child. This makes sense if you think about it. How are you able to fully care for someone else if you do not care for yourself? I highly suggest that you not put off the self-care part of your life as you will soon burn yourself out.

Regardless of what self-care looks like for you, do it regularly! For me, personally, I am very sensitive to others' energy, and seeing up to 27 patients in a single day (plus the charting, phone calls, refills, tasks, and labs) can be as exhausting mentally as physically. I know that at the end of a long week of seeing patients I need to do something fun and/or relaxing to replenish my spent energy. I found that a Friday night restorative yoga class is just what I need to bring me back into balance.

You know yourself better than anyone else, so I suggest doing things that you enjoy to care for yourself. Whether this be a weekly massage, dancing with friends, yoga classes, or a dinner out with loved ones, taking care of yourself is essential to taking care of your patients. And as the infamous Tom Haverford from *Parks and Recs* would say, "TREAT YO'SELF!"

Regularly Schedule Time Off

My former medical director once shared a piece of advice she had heard from another provider. The suggestion was to schedule time off every three months to avoid getting burned out. Now depending on where you work, this may not be a viable option; however, I do agree with the idea of regular breaks, and every three months seems to be a good timeline for this. Maybe once you start working you'll find that you need a long weekend every two months or perhaps a week off every four months. Whatever the length may be, I highly suggest you try out this system. Taking time off allows you to replenish your batteries and to rejuvenate. You'll feel much more refreshed going back to work after some much needed and deserved time off.

Stay Connected with Your Nurse Practitioner Friends

A day without laughter is a day wasted.

—Charlie Chaplin

As often as I can, I try to catch up with my nurse practitioner friends for dinner or a phone call. During this time, we catch up with each other's lives and also relate patient stories (all HIPAA compliant, of course!). I remember one time, the four of us were at a Mexican restaurant discussing intramuscular injections into the buttock. We were discussing how to avoid hitting the sciatic nerve and the best technique for this. One of my friends (the most experienced of the group) proceeded to get up and draw a cross over her right buttock to demonstrate this marker. She squeezed her flesh, avidly pointing to us that *this* was the safest spot where you should inject. We were all cracking up because in what other profession can you do this (without thinking anything is out of the ordinary) while eating guacamole and chips in a restaurant full of people?

I have many memories of such moments, laughing with friends over a funny patient interaction or discussing how to better manage a patient I had seen. These NP friends are in the trenches with me and always have my back. I adore them for all of their encouragement when I succeed and all their support when I fail. They know what the daily life of an NP is like and are always there to lend an ear if needed. I encourage each and every one of you to maintain relationships like these where you can laugh through some of life's most challenging moments. These are the people who understand exactly what you have been through, both the peaks and the valleys. Keep in touch with your NP friends. I can't imagine what I'd do without mine; they truly have become like family to me.

———

As you have seen from this chapter, working as a nurse practitioner can come with a lot of stressors. From managing and caring for sick patients to all of the other on-the-job responsibilities being tossed at you, life as an NP at times can be challenging. Nevertheless, it is my firm belief that if you are successfully able to manage the influx of work being tossed at you, and have a little fun at the same time, you will set yourself up for a successful and rewarding career as a nurse practitioner.

Don't forget that taking care of yourself is just as important as taking care of your patients. Spend time outside of work doing the things you love and spend time with those you love the most. Hopefully at the end of the day the work you are doing and the people you are helping will outweigh all the challenges that come with the territory. I have found that by focusing on the patients I helped, and not the ones who were complaining or angry, helps to put things into perspective. Remember, life is a journey, and it's best to enjoy the ride.

EPILOGUE

Now this is not the end. It's not even the beginning of the end. But it is perhaps the end of the beginning.

—Winston Churchill

The day that my official New York state prescription pads arrived in the mail was bittersweet. I had just started a job at a nurse practitioner–run primary care clinic and had been eagerly awaiting my personalized prescription pad for months. As I opened the package and pulled out the two pads, each with one hundred personalized scripts, I marveled at just how far I had come. It was almost three and a half years since my very first day of nursing school, and six years since I took my first prerequisite course. So much had happened between then and now, and I couldn't believe that I was actually looking at an official prescription pad with my name and title on it.

Although I was in complete awe, unfortunately two of the people I'd always wanted to send a handwritten prescription, my dad and my grandmother, had both passed away within the previous six months. I had so badly wanted to send them each a personalized prescription, and I held back tears knowing that I never would be able to do so.

The pad was symbolic in that it was a testament to all that I had endured to get to that moment: the countless hours that I had spent putting into my numerous clinical rotations, studying for exams, endless paperwork for licensing and certifications, and so much more. And yet here I was—a board certified New York State licensed nurse practitioner with prescriptive authority. Although my father and grandmother would never get their very own prescription written by me, they had been with me throughout my journey, and continue to be with me on some other plane in time and space. I know wherever they are, they are proud of what I have done and accomplished.

It is my sincerest wish that this book has been able to help you on your life path, whether it is to become a nurse practitioner or not. Perhaps this book made you realize becoming an NP was not right for you, thus pointing you in the correct direction. Or maybe something you read within the pages re-emphasized the importance of following your NP dream. Regardless of where you are in your journey to become a nurse practitioner, I wish you great success and happiness in all that you do.

APPENDIX

The following pages provide an extensive list of references to guide you on your nurse practitioner career. The list includes board certifying organizations, references to help you finance your education, job search resources, and academic references to help you throughout your nurse practitioner program and professional career.

I've grouped resources by general subheading; however, some of these websites have multiple resources available besides the heading I've listed them under. You will also notice that some organizations are listed more than once as I've found additional information that I felt was valuable to the reader.

This list is by no means all-inclusive. I encourage you to continue searching other websites and resources for more updated and supplemental information. Additionally, this information provided was correct at the time of publication and may have changed since. Please refer to individual websites for the most up-to-date information. I have not been paid to promote any organization below and have found the resources through my own individual research or from discussions with colleagues.

Board Certification Organizations

As stated earlier in the text, to become board certified in a certain specialty or subspecialty you need to take the certification examination. Different organizations offer different examinations, and you will need to find the organization that best fits your specialty. This list may not be all-inclusive, and I encourage you to do additional research if your specialty is not listed. At the time of publication of this book, the following specialty and subspecialty board examinations are being offered.

American Nurses Credentialing Center (ANCC) www.nursecredentialing.org

- Adult-Gerontology Acute Care NP
- Adult-Gerontology Primary Care NP
- Adult Psychiatric-Mental Health NP
- Family NP
- Pediatric Primary Care NP
- Psychiatric-Mental Health NP
- Emergency NP

The American Academy of Nurse Practitioners (AANP) www.aanpcert.org

- Adult-Gerontology Primary Care NP
- Family NP
- Emergency NP

American Holistic Nurses Certification Corporation www.ahncc.org

- Advanced Practice Holistic Nurse (APHN-BC)

The Dermatology Nurses Association www.dnanurse.org

- Dermatology Certified Nurse Practitioner

The Hospice and Palliative Credentialing Center www.hpna.org

- Advanced Certified Hospice and Palliative Nurse (ACHPN)

The National Certification Corporation www.nccwebsite.org

- Neonatal Nurse Practitioner
- Women's Health Care Nurse Practitioner

The Oncology Nursing Certification Organization (ONCC) www.oncc.org

- Advanced Oncology Certified Nurse Practitioner

The Pediatric Nursing Certification Board www.pncb.org

- Certified Pediatric Nurse Practitioner—Acute Care
- Certified Pediatric Nurse Practitioner—Primary Care

Wound Ostomy and Continence Nursing Certification Board www.wocncb.
org

- Wound Care
- Ostomy Care
- Continence Care

Academic Websites and Journals

The list below includes some of the websites that I've used for research purposes or to learn more about a certain topic. Many of the sites have been
incredibly helpful when looking for information on how to best treat a patient.
The list is not specific to nurse practitioners, and as you will see the majority
of the websites listed belong to other medical professions. Nevertheless, they
can be used by clinicians from a variety of healthcare specialties and will be
beneficial to the NP, including those in specialty practice.

A few of these websites and journals are also very useful as they have the
most up-to-date guidelines. Additionally, many sites have information regarding conferences, CEs, and how to get involved with your peers. They may also
be used as patient education tools and can guide patients looking to connect
with providers and resources.

Regardless of your specialty, you may find these resources beneficial, and I
encourage you to read through the list. This list is by no means all-inclusive, and
I encourage you to continue to your scholarly resources.

- Academy of Neonatal Nursing www.academyonline.org
- Advance for Nurse Practitioners
  http://nurse-practitioners-and-physician-assistants.advanceweb.com/
- American Academy of Allergy & Asthma and Immunology www.
  aaaai.org

- American Academy of Clinical Oncology www.asco.org
- American Academy of Dermatology www.aad.org
- American Academy of Emergency Medicine www.aaem.org
- American Academy of Family Physicians www.aafp.org
- American Academy of Hospice and Palliative Medicine www.aahpm.org
- American Academy of Ophthalmology www.aao.org
- American Academy of Orthopedic Surgeons www.aaos.org
- American Academy of Otolaryngology—Head and Neck Surgery www.entnet.org
- American Academy of Pediatrics www.aap.org
- American College of Cardiology www.acc.org
- American College of Emergency Physicians www.acep.org
- The American College of Physicians www.acponline.org
- American College of Rheumatology www.rheumatology.org
- The American Congress of Obstetricians and Gynecologists www.acog.org
- American Journal of Nursing http://journals.lww.com/ajnonline/pages/default.aspx
- American Journal of Epidemiology https://academic.oup.com/aje
- The American Journal of Medicine www.amjmed.com
- American Psychiatric Association www.psychiatry.org
- American Society for Metabolic and Bariatric Surgery www.asmbs.org
- The American Society of Hematology www.hematology.org
- The American Society of Pediatric Hematology/Oncology www.aspho.org
- American Society of Plastic Surgeons www.plasticsurgery.org
- Clinical Advisor http://www.clinicaladvisor.com
- Clinician Reviews http://www.mdedge.com/clinicianreviews
- Family Practice Notebook www.fpnotebook.com
- Immunization Action Coalition (IAC) www.immunize.org
- The Infectious Diseases Society of America www.idsociety.org
- The International Society of Travel Medicine www.istm.org
- Journal of the American Academy of Dermatology www.jaad.org
- The Journal of Emergency Medicine www.jem-journal.com
- The Journal for Nurse Practitioners http://www.npjournal.org
- Journal of Pediatric Health Care http://www.jpedhc.org
- Journal of Urgent Care Medicine www.jucm.com

- The New England Journal of Medicine http://www.nejm.org
- The Nurse Practitioner http://journals.lww.com/tnpj/pages/default.aspx
- NutritionFacts.org www.nutritionfacts.org
- The Physicians Committee for Responsible Medicine www.pcrm.org
- Physicians for Social Responsibility www.psr.org
- Society for Academic Emergency Medicine www.saem.org
- Travel Medicine and Infectious Disease www.travelmedicinejournal.com
- UpToDate www.uptodate.com

Scholarship Websites and Financing Your Education

The list below consists of scholarship and financial aid resources in addition to those mentioned in chapter four. Remember that your school will most likely have multiple in-house scholarships/additional financial aid that you can apply for as well. Additionally, there are state-specific scholarships. Make sure to do your research to determine if additional funding is available to you.

- After College Scholarship Fund https://www.aftercollege.com/content/article/aftercollege-aacn-scholarship
- American Association of Colleges of Nursing http://www.aacnnursing.org
- American Association of Nurse Practitioners http://www.aanp.org/practice/grants-scholarships2
- Bigfuture https://bigfuture.collegeboard.org
- Cappex www.cappex.com
- College Grants www.collegegrants.org
- College Scholarships www.collegescholarships.org
- Daughters of the American Revolution https://www.dar.org/national-society/scholarships#nursing
- Discover Nursing www.discovernursing.com/scholarships
- Doctors of Nursing Practice http://www.doctorsofnursingpractice.org/resources/grants-and-scholarships/
- Explore Health Careers http://explorehealthcareers.org/en/home
- Fastweb http://www.fastweb.com/
- Fedmoney www.fedmoney.org
- Finaid www.finaid.org

- GoodCall https://www.goodcall.com/scholarships/
- Health Wonk Scholarship https://www.healthinsurance.org/scholarship/
- HRSA www.hrsa.gov
- International Financial Aid and College Scholarship Search http://www.iefa.org
- Jeannette Rankin Women's Scholarship Fund www.rankinfoundation.org
- Johnson & Johnson—The Campaign for Nursing's Future http://www.discovernursing.com
- Kentucky Coalition of Nurse Practitioners & Nurse Midwives http://www.kcnpnm.org/?page=scholarship
- Minute Clinic Scholarship http://www.cvs.com/minuteclinic/resources/jj-together-we-care
- The National Association of Pediatric Nurse Practitioners Foundation www.napnapfoundation.org
- Native Hawaiian Health Scholarship https://bhw.hrsa.gov/loansscholarships/nhhs
- Nurse Journal http://nursejournal.org/articles/nursing-scholarships-grants
- Nursing Scholarships www.nursingscholarships.org
- The Nurse Practitioner Healthcare Foundation https://www.nphealthcarefoundation.org
- Nursing Scholarship http://www.nursingscholarship.us
- Oncology Nursing Society Foundation www.onsfoundation.org
- Point Foundation, The National LGBTQ Scholarship Fund www.pointfoundation.org
- Scholarship Owl www.scholarshipowl.com
- Scholarship Points www.scholarshippoints.com
- Tylenol Future Care Scholarship http://www.tylenol.com/news/scholarship
- Unigo www.unigo.com

National and International Nursing and Nurse Practitioner Organizations

Below is a list of national and international nursing and nurse practitioner organizations. Many of these organizations offer a plethora of resources such as job postings, continuing education units, conferences, and scholarship opportunities.

- Academy of Oncology Nurse and Patient Navigators www.aonnon line.org
- Advanced Practice Provider Executives www.appexecutives.org
- Advanced Practitioner Society for Hematology and Oncology www. apsho.org
- American Academy of Emergency Nurse Practitioners (AAENP) http:// aaenp-natl.org
- American Association of Colleges of Nursing www.aacnnursing.org
- American Association of Critical-Care Nurses (AACN) www.aacn. org
- American Association of Neuroscience Nurses www.aann.org
- American Association of Nurse Practitioners (AANP) www.aanp.org
- American Association for Men in Nursing www.aamn.org
- American Board of Nursing Specialties (ABNS) www.nursingcertifica tion.org
- American College of Nurse-Midwives www.midwife.org
- American Holistic Nurses Association www.ahna.org
- American Nurses Association (ANA) www.nursingworld.org
- American Nurse Practitioners Foundation www.anpf-foundation.org
- American Psychiatric Nurses Association (APNA) www.apna.org
- American Travel Health Nurses Association www.athna.org
- Asian American/Pacific Islander Nurses Association Inc. www.aapina. org
- Association of Advanced Practice Psychiatric Nurses www.aappn.org
- Association of Camp Nursing www.campnurse.org
- Association of Faculties of Pediatric Nurse Practitioners http://www. afpnp.org
- The Association of Occupational Health Nurse Practitioners (UK) www.aohnp.co.uk
- Association of Nurse Practitioners in Business, Inc. www.anpbfl.org
- Australian College of Nurse Practitioners www.acnp.org.au
- Dermatology Nurses Association www.dnanurse.org
- Doctors of Nursing Practice www.doctorsofnursingpractice.org
- Emergency Nurses Association www.ena.org
- Exceptional Nurse www.exceptionalnurse.com
- Gerontological Advanced Practice Nurses Association (GAPNA) www. gapna.org
- International Council of Nurses www.icn.ch

- International Council of Nurse Practitioners https://international. aanp.org
- National Academy of Dermatology Nurse Practitioners www.nadnp. net
- National Association of Hispanic Nurses www.nahnnet.org
- National Association of Neonatal Nurses www.nann.org
- National Association of Orthopaedic Nurses www.orthonurse.org
- National Association of Pediatric Nurse Practitioners (NAPNAP) www. napnap.org
- National Black Nurse Practitioner Association https://nbnpa.enpnet work.com
- National Coalition of Ethnic Minority Nurse Associations www. ncemna.org
- National Council of State Boards of Nursing www.ncsbn.org
- National Nurse Practitioner Symposium www.npsymposium.com
- National Nurses United www.nationalnursesunited.org
- National Organization of Nurse Practitioner Faculties www.nonpf.org
- New England Association of Neonatal Nurses www.neann.org
- Nurses International www.nursesinternational.org
- Nurse Practitioner Associates for Continuing Education (NPACE) www.npace.org
- Nurse Practitioner Association of Canada www.npac-aiipc.org
- Nurse Practitioners in Women's Health www.npwh.org
- NursingLicensure.org www.nursinglicensure.org
- Nursys www.nursys.com
- Oncology Nursing Society www.ons.org
- Philippine Nurses Association, Inc. www.pna-ph.org
- Preventative Cardiovascular Nurses Association www.pcna.net

State Nurse and Nurse Practitioner Organizations

For the following list, I've tried to include each state's nurse practitioner association and nursing organization as well as the state board of nursing website. You'll see that some states have multiple nursing and nurse practitioner organizations. I've also included state-specific scholarships and loan repayment opportunities in this section.

- **Alabama**

  Advanced Practitioners for the River Region https://riverregionap. enpnetwork.com

  Alabama Association of Nursing Students http://www.alabamanursing students.org

  Alabama Board of Nursing www.abn.alabama.gov

  Alabama Scholarships and Loans www.abn.alabama.gov/scholarships

  Alabama State Nurses Association www.alabamanurses.org

  Bay Area Nurse Practitioner Association https://banpa.enpnetwork.com

  Central Alabama Nurse Practitioner Association https://canpa.enpnet work.com

  North Alabama Nurse Practitioner Association https://northalabam anpa.enpnetwork.com

  Nurse Practitioner Alliance of Alabama https://npalliancealabama. enpnetwork.com

  West Alabama Nurse Practitioners https://wanp.enpnetwork.com

- **Alaska**

  Alaska Board of Nursing https://www.commerce.alaska.gov/web/cbpl/ ProfessionalLicensing/BoardofNursing

  Alaska Nurses Association www.aknurse.org

  Alaska Nurse Practitioner Association https://anpa.enpnetwork.com

  National Alaska Native American Indian Nurses Association www. nanainanurses.com

- **Arizona**

  Arizona Cannabis Nurse's Association www.azcna.com

  Arizona Emergency Nurses Association www.azena.org

  Arizona Nurses Association www.aznurse.org

  Arizona Nurse Practitioner Council https://arizonanp.enpnetwork.com

  Arizona State Board of Nursing https://www.azbn.gov

  Black Nurses Association Greater Phoenix Area www.bnaphoenix.org

  Coalition of Arizona Nurses in Advanced Practice http://aznpconnec tion.netfirms.com

  The National Association of Hispanic Nurses: Phoenix Chapter www. nahn-phx.org

  Philippine Nurses Association of Arizona www.pnaaz.org

  School Nurses Organization of Arizona www.snoa.org

- **Arkansas**
  Arkansas School Nurses Association https://asna.nursingnetwork.com
  Arkansas State Board of Nursing www.arsbn.org
  Arkansas State Board of Nursing Loans & Scholarships www.arsbn.org/loans-scholarships
  Arkansas Nurses Association www.arna.org
  Arkansas Nurse Practitioner Association https://anpassociation.enpnetwork.com

- **California**
  American Nurses Association/California www.anacalifornia.org
  Bay Area Nurse Practitioner Association https://banpa.enpnetwork.com
  The California Association for Nurse Practitioners www.canpweb.org
  California Board of Registered Nursing www.rn.ca.gov
  California State Loan Repayment Program www.oshpd.ca.gov/hwdd/slrp.html
  Northern California Chapter of GAPNA https://nccgapna.enpnetwork.com
  Orange County NAPNAP Chapter https://ocnapnap.enpnetwork.com
  Redding Area PA & NP Alliance https://rapanpa.enpnetwork.com

- **Colorado**
  Colorado Nurses Association www.coloradonurses.org
  Colorado Board of Nursing www.colorado.gov/pacific/dora/Nursing
  Colorado Health Service Corps www.colorado.gov/pacific/cdphe/colorado-health-service-corps
  The Colorado Society of Advanced Practice Nursing https://csapn.enpnetwork.com
  The Northern Colorado Nurse Practitioner Coalition https://ncnpc.enpnetwork.com
  The Southern Colorado Advanced Practice Nurses Association https://scapna.enpnetwork.com

- **Connecticut**
  Connecticut Advanced Practice Registered Nurse Society https://ctaprns.enpnetwork.com
  Connecticut Nurses Association www.ctnurses.org
  Department of Public Health Registered Nurse Licensure http://www.ct.gov/dph/cwp/view.asp?a=3121&q=389432

- **Delaware**
  Delaware Board of Nursing http://dpr.delaware.gov/boards/nursing/
  Delaware Coalition of Nurse Practitioners https://dcnpweb.enpnet work.com
  Delaware Nurses Association www.denurses.org

- **District of Columbia**
  Department of Health, Board of Nursing
  https://doh.dc.gov/lpn-application-package
  District of Columbia Nurses Association www.dcna.org
  Nurse Practitioner Association of the District of Columbia https://npadc.enpnetwork.com

- **Florida**
  Central Florida Advanced Nursing Practice Council https://cfanpc.enpnetwork.com
  Florida Association of Nurse Practitioners www.flanp.org
  Florida Board of Nursing http://floridasnursing.gov
  Florida Nurses Association www.floridanurse.org
  Florida Nurse Practitioner Network https://fnpn.enpnetwork.com
  Florida Panhandle Nurse Practitioner Coalition https://fpnpc.enpnet work.com
  North Central Florida Advanced Practice Nurses https://ncfapn.enp network.com/
  Nurse Practitioner Council of Collier County https://npccolliercounty.enpnetwork.com
  Nurse Practitioner Council of Miami-Dade https://npmiami.enpnet work.com
  Nurse Practitioner Council of Palm Beach County https://npcouncil pbc.enpnetwork.com
  PAs and NPs of the Florida Keys https://panpfloridakeys.enpnetwork.com/
  Polk County Advanced Practice Nurses Association www.pcapna.org
  South Florida Council of Advanced Practice Nurses. https://sfcapn.enpnetwork.com
  Tallahassee Area Council of Advanced Practice Nurses https://cap ntally.enpnetwork.com/
  Tampa Bay Advanced Practice Nurses Council https://tbapnc.enpnet work.com

- **Georgia**
  Central Georgia Advanced Practice Registered Nurses https://cgaprn.enpnetwork.com
  Georgia Board of Nursing http://sos.ga.gov/index.php/licensing/plb/45
  Georgia Nurses Association www.georgianurses.org
  South Georgia Association of Nurse Practitioners-Valdosta https://vuaprn.enpnetwork.com
  United Advanced Practice Registered Nurses of Georgia https://uaprn.enpnetwork.com

- **Hawaii**
  American Organization of Nurse Executives Hawaii www.aonehawaii.org
  Department of Commerce and Consumer Affairs Professional and Vocational Licensing http://cca.hawaii.gov/pvl/boards/nursing
  Hawaii Nurses Association www.hawaiinurses.org
  The Hawaii State Loan Repayment Program https://www.ahec.hawaii.edu/loan/

- **Idaho**
  Idaho Board of Nursing http://ibn.idaho.gov/IBNPortal/
  Idaho Nurses Association www.idahonurses.org
  Idaho State Loan Repayment Program http://healthandwelfare.idaho.gov
  Intermountain Advanced Practice Nurses Association https://iapna.enpnetwork.com
  Nurse Practitioners of Idaho www.npidaho.org

- **Illinois**
  Chicago Chapter of NAPNAP https://chicagonapnap.enpnetwork.com
  Illinois Department of Financial & Professional Regulation (IDFPR) http://www.idfpr.com/profs/nursing.asp
  Illinois Center for Nursing http://nursing.illinois.gov
  Illinois Center for Nursing, Financial Aid, Scholarships and Grants http://nursing.illinois.gov/financial.asp#INSTFUND
  Illinois Nurses Association www.illinoisnurses.com
  Illinois Society for Advanced Practice Nursing www.isapn.org

- **Indiana**
  Coalition of Advanced Practice Nurse of Indiana http://www.capni.org/
  Indiana State Board of Nursing http://www.in.gov/pla/nursing.htm
  Indiana State Nurses Association www.indiananurses.org
  Society of Nurses in Advanced Practice www.snapaprn.org

- **Iowa**
  Iowa Association of Nurse Practitioners https://iowaanp.enpnetwork.com/
  Iowa Nurse Practitioner Society www.iowanpsociety.org
  Iowa Board of Nursing https://nursing.iowa.gov/
  Iowa Loan Repayment Program
  https://idph.iowa.gov/ohds/rural-health-primary-care/primecarre
  Iowa Nurses Association http://portals7.gomembers.com/iowanurses/Home.aspx

- **Kansas**
  4 State APN www.4stateapn.org
  Kansas Advanced Practice Nurses Association https://kapn.enpnetwork.com
  Kansas Alliance of Advanced Nurse Practitioners www.kaanpks.com
  Kansas Nursing Association www.ksnurses.com
  Kansas State Board of Nursing http://www.ksbn.org/
  Northeast Kansas Nurse Practitioner Alliance https://kansasnps.enpnetwork.com

- **Kentucky**
  Kentucky Board of Nursing http://kbn.ky.gov
  Kentucky Coalition of Nurse Practitioners & Nurse Midwives www.kcnpnm.org
  Kentucky Nurses Association www.kentucky-nurses.org

- **Louisiana**
  Louisiana Association of Nurse Practitioners https://lanp.enpnetwork.com/
  Louisiana State Board of Nursing www.lsbn.state.la.us
  Louisiana State Loan Repayment Program http://dhh.louisiana.gov/index.cfm/page/1195
  Louisiana State Nurses Association www.lsna.org

- **Maine**
  Finance Authority of Maine www.famemaine.com
  Maine Nurse Practitioner Association www.mnpa.us
  Maine State Board of Nursing http://maine.gov/boardofnursing/
  The American Nurses Association-Maine www.anamaine.org

- **Maryland**
  Maryland Academy of Advanced Practice Clinicians
  https://maapconline.enpnetwork.com
  Maryland Board of Nursing http://mbon.maryland.gov
  Maryland Nurses Association www.marylandrn.org
  Nurse Practitioner Association of Maryland www.npamonline.org

- **Massachusetts**
  Massachusetts Board of Registration in Nursing www.mass.gov/eohhs/
  gov/departments/dph/programs/hcq/dhpl/nursing/
  Massachusetts Coalition of Nurse Practitioners www.mcnpweb.org
  Massachusetts Loan Repayment Program
  www.mass.gov/how-to/apply-for-the-massachusetts-loan-repay
  ment-program
  Massachusetts Nursing Association www.massnurses.org

- **Michigan**
  Great Lakes Chapter of GAPNA https://glcgapna.enpnetwork.com
  Michigan Board of Nursing www.michigan.gov
  Michigan Council of Nurse Practitioners www.micnp.org/index.html
  Michigan League for Nursing www.michleaguenursing.org
  Michigan Nurses Association www.minurses.org
  Michigan State Loan Repayment Program www.michigan.gov

- **Minnesota**
  Association of Southeastern Minnesota Nurse Practitioners
  https://asmnp.enpnetwork.com/
  Minnesota APRN Coalition https://mnaprnc.enpnetwork.com
  Minnesota Board of Nursing https://mn.gov/boards/nursing/
  Minnesota Health Care Loan Forgiveness Program
  www.health.state.mn.us/divs/orhpc/funding/loans/index.html
  Minnesota Nurses Association www.mnnurses.org
  Minnesota Nurse Practitioners www.mnnp.org
  Minnesota Organization of Registered Nurses www.mnorn.org

School Nurses Association of Minnesota www.minnesotaschoolnurses.org

- **Mississippi**
  Forgivable Loan Repayment Program
  http://riseupms.com/state-aid/loanscholarship-repayment-information
  Mississippi Association of Nurse Practitioners www.msanp.org
  Mississippi Board of Nursing www.msbn.ms.gov
  Mississippi Nurses Association www.msnurses.org

- **Missouri**
  Advanced Practice Nurses of the Ozarks www.apno.net
  Association of Missouri Nurse Practitioners https://amnp.enpnetwork.com/
  Missouri Division of Professional Registration-Board of Nursing
  http://pr.mo.gov/nursing.asp
  Missouri Nurses Association www.missourinurses.org

- **Montana**
  Montana Board of Nursing http://boards.bsd.dli.mt.gov/nur
  Montana Nurses Association www.mtnurses.org

- **Nebraska**
  Nebraska Department of Health and Human Services
  http://dhhs.ne.gov/publichealth/pages/crlNursingHome.aspx
  Nebraska Nurses Association www.nebraskanurses.org
  Nebraska Nurse Practitioners www.nebraskanp.org

- **Nevada**
  Nevada Advanced Practice Nurses Association https://napna.enpnetwork.com
  Nevada Nurses Association www.nvnurses.org
  Nevada State Board of Nursing www.nevadanursingboard.org

- **New Hampshire**
  New Hampshire Nurses Association www.nhnurses.org
  New Hampshire Board of Nursing www.oplc.nh.gov/nursing
  New Hampshire Nurse Practitioner Association https://nhnpa.enpnetwork.com

- **New Jersey**
  Advanced Practice Nurses of New Jersey www.apn-nj.org
  New Jersey Board of Nursing www.njconsumeraffairs.gov/nur
  New Jersey State Nurses Association www.njsna.org

- **New Mexico**
  Lea County Nurse Practitioners www.lcnpg.org
  New Mexico Board of Nursing http://nmbon.sks.com
  New Mexico Emergency Nurses Association www.nmena.org
  New Mexico Native American Indian Nurses Association www.nmnaina.org
  New Mexico Nurses Association www.nmna.org
  New Mexico Nurse Practitioner Council www.nmnpc.org

- **New York**
  New York State Nurses Association www.nysna.org
  The Nurse Practitioner Association-New York State www.thenpa.org
  Nurse Practitioner Association-New York State-Long Island Chapter www.npali.org
  Office of the Professions, Nursing www.op.nysed.gov/prof/nurse

- **North Carolina**
  Metrolina Coalition of Nurse Practitioners www.metrolinanp.org
  NCNA Council of Nurse Practitioners Wake/Central Region https://ncnpcouncil.enpnetwork.com
  NC Board of Nursing www.ncbon.com
  North Carolina Nurses Association www.ncnurses.org

- **North Dakota**
  North Dakota Board of Nursing www.ndbon.org
  North Dakota Nurses Association www.ndna.org
  North Dakota Nurse Practitioner Association http://nprac.nd.associationcareernetwork.com

- **Ohio**
  Northeast Ohio Nurse Practitioners www.neonp.org
  Ohio Association of Advanced Practice Nurses www.oaapn.org
  Ohio Chapter of GAPNA www.ohiogapna.org
  Ohio Nurses Association www.ohnurses.org
  Ohio Nurses Foundation www.ohionursesfoundation.org
  State of Ohio Board of Nursing www.nursing.ohio.gov

- **Oklahoma**
  Association of Oklahoma Nurse Practitioners www.npofoklahoma.com
  Oklahoma Board of Nursing www.nursing.ok.gov
  Oklahoma Nurses Association www.oklahomanurses.org

- **Oregon**
  Nurse Practitioners of Oregon www.nursepractitionersoforegon.org
  Oregon Holistic Nurses Association www.oregonholisticnurses.org
  Oregon Nurses Association www.oregonrn.org
  Oregon State Board of Nursing www.oregon.gov/osbn

- **Pennsylvania**
  BuxMont Nurse Practitioner Group https://buxmontnp.enpnetwork.com
  Chesmont Nurse Practitioner and Physician Assistant Association www.chesmontnppa.org
  Nurse Practitioners of Central Pennsylvania https://npcp.enpnetwork.com
  Nurse Practitioners of Northeastern Pennsylvania, LLC www.npnepa.org
  Pennsylvania Coalition of Nurse Practitioners www.pacnp.org
  Pennsylvania Delaware Valley NAPNAP www.padelvalnapnap.org
  Pennsylvania State Nurses Association www.psna.org
  State Board of Nursing www.dos.pa.gov/ProfessionalLicensing/BoardsCommissions/Nursing
  Student Nurses' Association of Pennsylvania www.snap-online.org

- **Rhode Island**
  Rhode Island State Nurses Association www.risna.org
  Nurse Practitioner Alliance of Rhode Island https://npari.enpnetwork.com
  State of Rhode Island Department of Health www.health.ri.gov/licenses

- **South Carolina**
  South Carolina Nurses Association www.scnurses.org
  South Carolina Board of Nursing www.llr.state.sc.us/pol/nursing
  Upstate Nurse Practitioner Association www.upstatenursepractitioner.com

- **South Dakota**
  Nurse Practitioner Association of South Dakota https://npasd.enpnet
  work.com
  South Dakota Board of Nursing https://doh.sd.gov/boards/nursing
  South Dakota Nurses Association www.sdnursesassociation.org

- **Tennessee**
  Chattanooga Area Nurses in Advanced Practice www.canap.org
  Board of Nursing https://tn.gov/health/topic/nursing-board
  Middle Tennessee Advanced Practice Nurses www.mtapn.org
  Northeast Tennessee Nurse Practitioners Association
  https://netnpa.enpnetwork.com
  Tennessee Nurses Association www.tnaonline.org
  Tennessee Nurse Practitioner Association https://tnnpa.enpnetwork.
  com
  West Tennessee Nurse Practitioners Alliance www.wtnpa.com

- **Texas**
  Austin Advanced Practice Nurses https://austinapns.enpnetwork.com
  Brazos Valley Nurse Practitioner Association www.bvnpa.org
  East Texas Nurse Practitioner Association www.etnpa.org
  Houston Area Chapter of NAPNAP www.houstonnapnap.org
  Houston Area Nurse Practitioners www.hanp.org
  North Harris Montgomery Advanced Practice Nurse Society
  www.nhmapns.com
  San Antonio Nurses in Advanced Practice www.sanap.org
  Texas Board of Nursing www.bon.texas.gov
  Texas Gulf Coast Chapter of GAPNA https://gcgapna.enpnetwork.
  com
  Texas Nurses Association www.texasnurses.org
  Texas Nurse Practitioners www.texasnp.org
  Valley Advanced Practice Nurse Association www.myvapna.org

- **Utah**
  Utah Chapter of NAPNAP www.utahnapnap.org
  Utah Division of Occupational and Professional Licensing, Nursing
  https://dopl.utah.gov/licensing/nursing.html
  Utah Nurses Association www.utnurse.org
  Utah Nurse Practitioners https://utahnp.enpnetwork.com

- **Vermont**
  American Nurses Association, Vermont www.ana-vermont.org
  Secretary of State, Nursing
  www.sec.state.vt.us/professional-regulation/list-of-professions/nursing
  The Vermont Nurse Practitioners Association www.vtnpa.org
  Vermont State School Nurses' Association www.vssna.org

- **Virginia**
  Virginia Board of Nursing www.dhp.virginia.gov/nursing
  Virginia Council of Nurse Practitioners www.vcnp.net
  Virginia Nurses Association www.virginianurses.com

- **Washington**
  ARNPs United of Washington State https://auws.enpnetwork.com
  Association of Advanced Practice Psychiatric Nurses www.aappn.org
  Association of Eastside Nurse Practitioners www.eastsidenp.org
  Loan Repayment www.wsac.wa.gov/health-professionals
  Mount Baker Nurse Practitioners Association www.mbnpa.org
  Nurse Practitioner Group of Spokane https://npgspokane.enpnetwork.com
  Puget Sound Nurse Practitioner Association www.psnpa.org
  Washington State Department of Health, Nurse Licensing
  www.doh.wa.gov/LicensesPermitsandCertificates/NursingCommission/NurseLicensing
  Washington State Nurses Association www.wsna.org

- **West Virginia**
  State Loan Repayment Program www.hsc.wvu.edu/icrh/financial-incentives/state-loan-repayment-program-slrp
  West Virginia RN Board of Nursing http://www.wvrnboard.wv.gov
  West Virginia Nurses Association www.wvnurses.org

- **Wisconsin**
  Board of Nursing
  https://dsps.wi.gov/Pages/RulesStatutes/Nursing.aspx
  Metro Milwaukee Nurse Practitioners
  https://metromilwaukeenp.enpnetwork.com
  Wisconsin Department of Health Services www.dhs.wisconsin.gov/primarycare/students.htm
  Wisconsin Nurses Association www.wisconsinnurses.org

- **Wyoming**
  Wyoming Council for Advanced Practice Nurses www.wcapn.org
  Wyoming Nurses Association www.wyonurse.org
  Wyoming State Board of Nursing https://nursing-online.state.wy.us

Jobs/Recruiting/Locum Tenens Organizations

- AANP Job Center https://jobcenter.aanp.org
- Academy Physicians www.academyphysicians.com
- Accountable Healthcare Staffing www.ahcstaff.com
- Addison Recruiting www.addisonhealth.com
- Advanced Practice www.advancedpractice.com
- Advanced Practice Solutions www.advancedpracticesolutions.com
- Advance Healthcare Network www.advanceweb.com
- Allied Health Search www.alliedhealthsearch.org
- All Medical Personnel www.allmedstaffing.com
- All Physician Jobs www.allphysicianjobs.com
- All Star Recruiting www.allstarrecruiting.com
- Aureus Medical Group www.aureusmedical.com
- Barton Associates www.bartonassociates.com
- BAS HealthCare www.bashealthcare.com
- CareerBuilder www.careerbuilder.com
- Catapult Physician Staffing www.catapultphysicians.com
- Club Staffing www.clubstaffing.com
- CompHealth www.comphealth.com
- Consilium Staffing www.consiliumstaffing.com
- Delta Locum Tenens www.deltalocums.com
- Doctor's Choice Placement Services www.doctorschoiceplacement.com
- Echo Locum Tenens www.echolocum.com
- Employment Crossing www.employmentcrossing.com
- ENP Network www.enpnetwork.com
- Ensearch Management Consultants-Neonatal NPs www.ensearch.com
- The Execu Search Group www.execu-search.com
- Fidelis Partners www.fidelismp.com
- FlexJobs www.flexjobs.com
- Floyd Lee Locums www.floydleelocums.com
- Glassdoor www.glassdoor.com
- GreenLife Healthcare Staffing www.glhstaffing.com

- Harris Medical Associates www.harrismedical.com
- Hayward DuPont www.haywarddupont.com
- Healthcare Employment Network www.healthcaretravelers.com
- Health eCareers www.healthecareers.com
- Health Jobs www.healthjobs.com
- Health Jobs Nationwide www.healthjobsnationwide.com
- Indeed www.indeed.com
- Infinity MedStaff www.infinitymedstaff.com
- Integrity Healthcare www.ihcrecruiting.com
- Integrity Locums www.ihcl.com
- Interim Physicians www.interimphysicians.com
- International Medical Placement www.intlmedicalplacement.com
- Jackson & Coker www.jacksoncoker.com
- Kendall & Davis www.kendallanddavis.com
- Locum Leaders www.locumleaders.com
- Locum Tenens www.locumtenens.com
- Loyal Source www.loyalsource.com
- Maxim Healthcare Services www.maximstaffing.com
- MD Staffers www.mdstaffers.com
- Medcare Staffing www.medcarestaffing.com
- MedeCareers www.medecareers.com
- Medical Advantage www.medicaladvantage.net
- Medical Doctor Associates www.mdainc.com
- Medical Recruiting www.medicalrecruiting.com
- Medical Search International www.medsearchint.com
- MEDPATH www.medpathjobs.com
- Merritt Hawkins www.merritthawkins.com
- Monster www.monster.com
- myMDcareers www.mymdcareers.com
- NAPNAP Career Connection http://careerconnection.napnap.org
- Nationwide Locum Tenens www.nationwidelocumtenens.com
- National Rural Recruitment and Retention Network (3Rnet) www.3rnet.org
- NEPRC www.neprc.com
- NP Canada www.npcanada.ca
- NP Jobs www.npjobs.com
- NP Now www.npnow.com
- NPPA Recruiters www.npparecruiters.com

- Nursing Job Cafe www.nursingjobcafe.com
- Odell Medical Search www.odellsearch.com
- One Path Career Partners www.onepathcareers.com
- One Stop Recruiting www.1stoprecruiting.com
- Oregon Nurse Career Center https://jobs.oregonrn.org
- PA Jobsite www.pajobsite.com
- PA and NP World www.panpworld.com
- Progressive Nursing Staffers www.progressivenursing.com
- Simply Hired www.simplyhired.com
- Smith & Associates Healthcare Placements www.panpjobs.com
- Source Medical www.source-medical.net
- Staff Care www.staffcare.com
- StaffMD www.staffmd.com
- Sunbelt Staffing www.sunbeltstaffing.com
- TalentDesk www.talentdesk.com
- Tal Healthcare www.talhealthcare.com
- Team Locums www.teamlocums.biz
- The Clinical Recruiter www.theclinicalrecruiter.com
- Ultimate Locum Tenens www.ultimatelt.com
- Velo Source www.velosource.com
- Virtus Placement www.virtusplacement.com
- Vista www.vistastaff.com
- Weatherby Healthcare www.weatherbyhealthcare.com
- Zip Recruiter www.ziprecruiter.com

Continuing Education Resources

There are a plethora of continuing education resources available for nurse practitioners. Many academic institutions offer continuing education conferences and it is best to check with each institution individually to see what conferences are available. Additionally, national medical organizations provide continuing education specific to their specialty. There are plenty more nurse practitioner CE resources aside from those listed below. This list is not all-inclusive so I encourage you to do a thorough search when looking into continuing education courses. Your state NP organization may offer CE as well.

- Advanced Practice Prep www.advancedpracticeprep.net
- American Association of Nurse Practitioners www.aanp.org/education/continuing-education-ce/ce-opportunities
- Barkley & Associates www.npcourses.com
- Continuing Education, Inc. www.continuingeducation.net
- NetCE http://www.netce.com/nursepractitioners
- Nurse Practitioner Associates for Continuing Education www.npace.org
- Mayo Clinic School of Continuous Professional Development www.ce.mayo.edu
- MDLinx www.mdlinx.com
- My CME www.mycme.com
- Practicing Clinicians Exchange www.practicingclinicians.com
- Prime www.primeinc.org
- TravelHealth101 www.travelhealth101.com